21st Century Sexualities

T0174133

A new "digital sexual revolution" is shaping the way we understand, experience, and live sexuality in the twenty-first century. The Internet, in particular, enables individuals and groups to learn about sexuality, experience their sexuality in new ways, create identities and sexual communities, and advocate for sexual rights and social justice.

Exploring this new era, *21st Century Sexualities* brings together more than fifty timely and accessible contributions to create a wide-ranging and compelling picture of contemporary American sexuality. Including a superb editorial overview, it incorporates the latest controversies, theory, and methodological material in the areas of:

- sexual literacy
- media and sexual commodification
- sexual health and wellness
- sexual rights and activism
- globalization.

Written by researchers and academics, as well as advocates and community-based practitioners, this lively and comprehensive collection is packed with cutting-edge research and advocacy material in sexuality studies. While it focuses on the US context, attention is given to global dimensions of sexuality, particularly its social and cultural aspects. It will appeal to undergraduates in women's and gender studies, anthropology and sociology, psychology and human development, contemporary media studies, and public health.

Gilbert Herdt, a cultural anthropologist, is Professor of Human Sexuality Studies and Anthropology and Director of Human Sexuality Studies at San Francisco State University, USA. He is also Director of the National Sexuality Resource Center.

Cymene Howe is Assistant Professor of Anthropology at American University, Washington, DC, USA.

21st Century Sexualities

Contemporary issues in health,
education, and rights

**Edited by
Gilbert Herdt and
Cymene Howe**

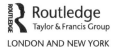
Routledge
Taylor & Francis Group

LONDON AND NEW YORK

First published 2007
by Routledge
2 Park Square, Milton Park, Abingdon, Oxon OX14 4RN

Simultaneously published in the USA and Canada
by Routledge
711 Third Avenue, New York, NY 10017, USA

Routledge is an imprint of the Taylor & Francis Group, an informa business

Typeset in Times New Roman by
Florence Production Ltd, Stoodleigh, Devon

British Library Cataloguing in Publication Data
A catalogue record for this book is available from the British Library

Library of Congress Cataloging in Publication Data
21st century sexualities: contemporary issues in health, education,
   and rights/edited by Gilbert Herdt and Cymene Howe.
      p. cm.
   Includes bibliographical references and index.
   1. Sex—Social aspects.   2. Sex—Social aspects—United States.
   3. Sexual ethics—United States.   4. Sex customs—United States.
   5. Sex instruction—United States.   6. Sexual minorities—United States.
   7. Hygiene, sexual—United States.   8. Sex—Computer network
   resources.   I. Herdt, Gilbert H., 1949–.   II. Howe, Cymene.
   III. Title: Twenty-first century sexualities.
   HQ16.A18 2007
   306.770973′090511—dc22   2006039007

ISBN10: 0–415–77306–7 (hbk)
ISBN10: 0–415–77307–5 (pbk)
ISBN10: 0–203–94747–9 (ebk)

ISBN13: 978–0–415–77306–5 (hbk)
ISBN13: 978–0–415–77307–2 (pbk)
ISBN13: 978–0–203–94747–0 (ebk)

Contents

Contributors

Genevieve Ames, Ph.D. received her doctorate in medical anthropology from the University of California at San Francisco and Berkeley. She is currently Adjunct Professor in the School of Public Health, University of California, Berkeley and Associate Director/Senior Scientist at the Pacific Institute for Research, Prevention Research Center.

Yorghos Apostolopoulos, Ph.D. is Visiting Professor of Social Epidemiology with the Cyprus International Institute/Harvard School of Public Health, Cyprus and Associate Clinical Professor of Medicine with the Emory University School of Medicine, USA. His work examines the ways social structure and the built environment affect health outcomes.

Andrew Bickford, Ph.D. is an Assistant Professor of Anthropology at George Mason University whose research centers on militarization, masculinity, public health, and post-socialist societies. He has received awards from the Fulbright Foundation and the Social Science Research Council and has a forthcoming book, *Red Radiation: The Cultural Politics of Militarized Citizenship in Germany*.

Lisa Cacari-Stone, Ph.D. is a W.K. Kellogg and Alonzo Yerby Post-Doctoral Scholar at the Harvard School of Public Health. Her research focuses on public policies as determinants of health for racial and ethnic populations in the southwest and Latino-heterogeneity in health status, access and service utilization.

Ann J. Cahill, Ph.D. is Associate Professor of Philosophy at Elon University. Her research interests include feminist theories of the body and social and political philosophy. She is the author of *Rethinking Rape* and is currently working on a critique of the feminist concept of objectification.

David Cameron, as a person with XXY sex chromosomes, has written about his experience in *Hermaphrodites with Attitude*, *Chrysalis*, and Alice Dreger's *Intersex in the Age of Ethics*. He is an appointed member to the San Francisco Human Rights Commission LGBT Advisory Committee and was a member of their Intersex Task Force.

Sealing Cheng, Ph.D. is Henry Luce Assistant Professor in the Women's Studies Department, Wellesley College. She researches issues of sexuality with a particular focus on sex work, migration, HIV/AIDS, and human rights. She is currently working on her manuscript *Transnational Desires: Filipina Entertainers in US Military Camp Towns in South Korea*.

David W. Coon, Ph.D. has conducted extensive research on issues of sexuality, aging and HIV, and has worked with the Institute on Aging in San Francisco.

Sonia Corrêa is the founder of SOS-Corpo, Gênero, Cidadania, a feminist non-governmental organization based in Recife, Brazil. Since 1992 she has been a member of DAWN (Development Alternative with Women for a New Era) as the coordinator for sexual reproductive health and rights.

Alberto Curotto, Ph.D. is a Research Analyst at the Center for AIDS Prevention Studies at University of California, San Francisco. In 2001, he began work on research projects to study gay men's Internet use and helped to design and evaluated web-based, HIV-prevention programs tailored for the sociocultural needs of gay men.

Bonnie Duran, Ph.D. is an Associate Professor in the Department of Family and Community Medicine at the University of New Mexico. Her research focuses on American Indian mental health and community-based participatory research.

Jessica Fields, Ph.D. is an Assistant Professor of Sociology at San Francisco State University and a Research Associate in the SFSU Center for Research on Gender and Sexuality. Her research explores the lessons students take from sex education about the intersections of sexuality, race, and gender inequalities.

Angel M. Foster, D.Phil., A.M. is an Associate at Ibis Reproductive Health and the 2003–2004 President of Medical Students for Choice.

Katherine Frank, Ph.D. is a cultural anthropologist, fiction writer, and former exotic dancer. She is the author of *G-Strings and Sympathy: Strip Club Regulars and Male Desire* and a co-editor of *Flesh for Fantasy: Producing and Consuming Exotic Dance*. She is currently researching how couples negotiate monogamy and writing an ethnography of erotic couples' tourism.

Gilberto R. Gerald, a Panamanian native and naturalized US citizen, is a 1974 Pratt Institute graduate in architecture. Since 1983 he has worked in the lesbian and gay rights movement and HIV/AIDS community-based work. He now supports these efforts through consulting work. His writing has appeared in several books and journals.

Adrienne Germain is President of the New York-based International Women's Health Coalition, which works to protect and promote the rights and health of girls and women worldwide. She was a member of US government delegations to United Nations conferences in the 1990s including the 1995 Fourth World Conference on Women, in Beijing.

Gloria González-López, Ph.D. is Assistant Professor of Sociology at the University of Texas at Austin. Born and raised in Monterrey, Mexico, she earned her Ph.D.

from the University of Southern California. Her book *Erotic Journeys: Mexican Immigrants and their Sex Lives* focuses on sexuality and immigration.

Jamison Green is a writer and educator specializing in transgender and transsexual health, safety, and civil rights, working internationally out of the San Francisco Bay Area. He transitioned from female to male in 1988 at the age of 40, and is the author of *Becoming a Visible Man*. For information, see www.jamisongreen.com.

Judith Halberstam, Ph.D. is Professor of English and Director of the Center for Feminist Research at University of Southern California. She is the author of *Skin Shows: Gothic Horror and the Technology of Monsters* and *Female Masculinity*, and co-author with Del LaGrace Volcano of *The Drag King Book* and *In a Queer Time and Place: Transgender Bodies, Subcultural Lives*.

Gilbert Herdt, Ph.D., a cultural anthropologist, is Professor of Human Sexuality Studies and Anthropology and Director of Human Sexuality Studies at San Francisco State University. Professor Herdt is also Director of the National Sexuality Resource Center, a Ford Foundation-funded project. To learn about NSRC's campaign for sexual literacy go to sexliteracy.org.

Paul Higate, D.Phil. is a Senior Lecturer in the Department of Politics at the University of Bristol in the UK. His main interest is the masculine culture of the military. He is currently researching perceptions and experiences of security in peacekeeping missions using the concepts of space and place.

Celeste Hirschman, M.A. is a researcher at the Center for Research on Gender and Sexuality and a certified sexological bodyworker.

Cymene Howe, Ph.D. is an Assistant Professor of Anthropology at American University whose research centers on social movements, subjectivity and sexuality in the US and Latin America. She was a Mellon Postdoctoral Fellow at Cornell University with a book forthcoming, *Erotiscapes: Sex, Social Justice and Nicaragua's New Media Era.*

Anthony Hunter, B.A. completed his undergraduate work in Speech and Communication at San Francisco State University and attended the graduate program in Rhetoric and Communication at the University of California, Davis.

Loraine Hutchins, Ph.D. teaches LGBT Studies, women's health and health issues in sexuality at the college level. She co-edited *Bi Any Other Name: Bisexual People Speak Out* and is one of the co-founders of the US bisexual liberation movement.

Janice M. Irvine, Ph.D. is a Professor of Sociology at the University of Massachusetts. She is also the Director of the Five College Women's Studies Research Center. Her most recent book is *Talk About Sex: The Battles Over Sex Education in the United States.*

Carole Joffe, Ph.D. is a Professor of Sociology at the University of California, Davis and a Visiting Professor at the Bixby Center for Reproductive Health Research and Policy at University of California, San Francisco. She is the author of *Doctors of Conscience: The Struggle to Provide Abortion before and after Roe v. Wade.*

Martha Kempner is the Associate Director of Information and Education of SIECUS, The Sexuality Information and Education Council of the United States. She oversees the activities of SIECUS's Community Advocacy Project including the monitoring, analysis, and reporting of trends in sexuality education, as well the activities of opponents of comprehensive sexuality education.

Robert M. Kertzner, M.D. is Associate Clinical Professor of Psychiatry at University of California, San Francisco and Adjunct Associate Research Scientist in the Department of Psychiatry, Columbia University. He has published in the areas of adult development and gay and lesbian mental health, sexuality in older adults and HIV and mental health.

Jennifer Kidwell is Communications Associate at the International Women's Health Coalition and a student at Columbia University's Mailman School of Public Health.

Jennie Kronenfeld, Ph.D. is Professor of Sociology in Arizona State University's School of Social and Family Dynamics. Her research is in medical sociology, health policy, health across the life course, health care utilization, and health behavior. She is editor of research for *Sociology of Health Care* and co-editor of *Health*.

Louise Lamphere, Ph.D. is a Distinguished Professor of Anthropology at the University of New Mexico. Her research focuses on gender and sexuality, women and work, and health care policy.

David M. Latini works at the University of California, San Francisco in the urology department.

Deborah Levine, M.A. is Executive Director of Internet Sexuality Information Services. Ms Levine has worked online for 12+ years, beginning with Columbia University's Go Ask Alice! She teaches "Sexuality and the Internet" at San Francisco State and is the author of *The Joy of Cybersex* and numerous academic papers.

Linwood J. Lewis, Ph.D. is Associate Professor of Psychology at Sarah Lawrence College and Adjunct Assistant Professor of Medical Psychology at Columbia University. His research interests range from development of sexuality in ethnic minority adolescents and adults to the effects of culture and social context on conceptualization of genetic health.

Rae Lewis, M.S., M.P.H., is a faculty member of Axia College of University of Phoenix. Her research focuses on public health problems among special populations and the ethics of research on people with serious mental illness.

Ann M. Lucas, J.D., Ph.D. earned her doctoral and Jurisprudence and Social Policy degrees at the University of California, Berkeley. She is currently Associate Professor in Justice Studies at San José State University. Her recent publications include "The Work of Sex Work" (Deviant Behavior) and "The Currency of Sex," in *Rethinking Commodification*.

Kris Scott Martí is a writer and researcher with a degree in Cultural Anthropology. She specializes in lesbian culture and has contributed to *Curve Magazine*, *Girlfriends*, *National Gay and Lesbian Review*, *San Francisco Bay Area Reporter*, and *American Sexuality*. She is a former editor for AfterEllen.com and currently blogs for Krisbeep.blogspot.com and AmericanSexuality.blogspot.com.

Rita M. Melendez, Ph.D. is Research Associate at the Center for Research on Gender and Sexuality and an Assistant Professor in Human Sexuality at San Francisco State University. She received her Ph.D. in Sociology from Yale University and a Master's Degree in Biostatistics from the Mailman School of Public Health at Columbia University.

Sandra E. Moore, M.D. is an Assistant Professor of Clinical Pediatrics at the Morehouse School of Medicine in Atlanta. She obtained her B.S. in Biochemistry and African American Studies, and received her Medical Degree from the University of Maryland Baltimore, completing her Pediatric Residency at the University of Maryland Medical Center.

Joyce Nishioka has received journalism awards for her writing on transgender issues and sexual stereotypes of Asian Americans in the media. She is the editor of *American Sexuality* magazine: americansexuality.org.

Christine E. Pettett is a Ph.D. candidate in anthropology at Yale University with research interests in sexuality, gender studies, public health, and public policy. Her doctoral dissertation addresses the role of political economic factors in social justice activism for lesbian and bisexual women in New Orleans, Louisiana.

Cynthia Pope, Ph.D. is an Assistant Professor of Geography and Women's Studies at Central Connecticut State University. Her research focuses on gender and health issues in the developing world. Her most recent work concentrates on HIV prevention and risk perception in the Caribbean area (Cuba, Jamaica, Belize) and Uganda.

Linda Prine, M.D. is a family physician at the Institute for Urban Family Health, and is on the faculty of the Beth Israel Residency Program in Urban Family Practice in New York City. She teaches abortion care and speaks at academic meetings on integrating abortion care into mainstream family practice.

Gregory Rebchook, Ph.D. is a researcher at University of California, San Francisco's Center for AIDS Prevention Studies. He is a sociocultural psychologist and has been working in HIV prevention since 1987. His current interests include HIV prevention for young gay/bisexual men and gay men's Internet use.

Jakob Rigi, Ph.D is an Assistant Professor in the Department of Anthropology at Cornell University and the author of *Post-Soviet Chaos: Violence and Dispossession* *in Kazakhstan.* He has published on the formation of the state, ethnicity, corruption, youth, and the relationship between the state and capital in Kazakhstan and Russia.

Christophe Robert, Ph.D. earned his doctorate at Cornell University and is a Postdoctoral Associate in the Council of Southeast Asia Studies and a Lecturer in the Department of Anthropology at Yale University. He has conducted ethnographic research in Saigon/Ho Chi Minh City, the Mekong Delta, and the city of Hue in central Vietnam.

Cynthia Rothschild has been a human rights and sexual rights activist for close to two decades. She is the Senior Policy Advisor for the Center for Women's Global Leadership, the author of *Written Out: How Sexuality is Used to Attack Women's Organizing* and other publications related to LGBT rights and HIV/AIDS. The article included in this collection was written when the author was the program officer in international policy at the International Women's Health Coalition in New York.

Ann Russ, Ph.D. is an Associate Research Scientist at the Prevention Research Center.

Stanton E. Samenow, Ph.D. is a Clinical Psychologist in Alexandria, Virginia. He is the author of *Inside the Criminal Mind* and *Before It's Too Late: Why Some Kids Get Into Trouble and What Parents Can Do About It.*

Russell P. Shuttleworth, Ph.D. is currently a Visiting Scholar at the Institute of Urban and Regional Planning, University of California, Berkeley, and a lecturer in the Human Sexuality Studies Program at San Francisco State University. Dr Shuttleworth's primary research and teaching interest is critical disability and sexuality studies.

Leslie Simon, Ph.D. chairs the Women's Studies Department at City College of San Francisco and coordinates Project SURVIVE, the campus sexual violence prevention program. Along with several community-based organizations, Project SURVIVE has recently launched Expect Respect SF, which intends to bring a healthy relationship program to all San Francisco high-school students.

Kathy Sisson serves on the Board of Directors for the Society for the Scientific Study of Sexuality and the Advisory Board for the Woodhull Freedom Foundation. She has published in the journals, *The Journal of Sex Research*, *Archives of Sexual Behavior*, *Sexualities*, and the *Lesbian and Gay Psychology Review*.

Donna Jo Smith, M.A. is a doctoral candidate in the Graduate Institute of Liberal Arts at Emory University and Research Associate in the Division of Infectious Diseases, Emory University School of Medicine, where she specializes in qualitative health research and gender and sexuality as they affect populations most at risk of HIV.

Sevil Sönmez is Associate Professor with the Cyprus College School of Business in Nicosia, Cyprus. Her research centers on the social psychological links between population mobility (leisure and occupational) and health.

Jennie Sparandara worked as Outreach Coordinator at the Access Project, an organization committed to strengthening community action, promoting social change, and improving health, especially for those who are most vulnerable.

Amy Sueyoshi, Ph.D. teaches classes on race, gender, and sexuality in Ethnic Studies and Human Sexuality Studies at San Francisco State University. She has published works on Asian America sexuality history, cross-dressing, and same-sex marriage. She is currently working on a manuscript on the intimate life of poet Yone Noguchi.

Juhu Thukral, J.D. is the Director of the Sex Workers Project at the Urban Justice Center. Her work on the legal concerns of sex workers combines her experience with economic justice, health, and safety issues among low-income women of color, particularly immigrants, and her work on sex workers' labor rights.

Leonore Tiefer, Ph.D. earned her doctorate in physiological psychology. She re-specialized as a clinical psychologist and has been affiliated with several New York City medical schools. She has a sex therapy practice and authored *Sex is Not a Natural Act and Other Essays*. In 2000 she began an educational campaign about medicalization: www.fsd-alert.org.

Tre Trefethen is a freelance writer in the Bay Area who has examined the divisions of sexuality in science, sports, and politics.

Jillian Todd Weiss, J.D. Ph.D. is Assistant Professor of Law and Society at Ramapo College. Her area of research is law and transgender issues. She is the author of journal articles on the subject and has consulted with many corporations on transgender policy, training, and customer communications strategies.

Tracy A. Weitz, PHD, MPA directs the Advancing New Standards in Reproductive Health Program of the Bixby Center for Reproductive Health Research and Policy at the University of California, San Francisco and serves as Associate Director for Public Policy at the University of California, San Francisco's National Center of Excellence in Women's Health.

Mariamne H. Whatley, Ph.D. is Professor of Women's Studies/Curriculum and Instruction, and Associate Dean in the School of Education at the University of Wisconsin-Madison. She writes about women's health and sexuality education. She co-authored with Elissa Henken, *Did You Hear About the Girl Who. . .?: Contemporary Legends, Folklore, and Human Sexuality*.

Renée T. White, Ph.D. is Professor of Sociology and Co-Director of Black Studies at Fairfield University. Her books include *Putting Risk in Perspective: Black Teenage Lives in the Era of AIDS* and the forthcoming *Globalization of HIV/AIDS: An Interdisciplinary Reader*. She co-edits the *Journal of HIV/AIDS Prevention in Children & Youth*.

Cathleen Willging, Ph.D. is a Research Scientist at the Behavioral Health Research Center of the Southwest, a division of the Pacific Institute for Research and Evaluation. Her research focuses on health care policy and the delivery of mental health services in rural settings.

Linda Williams, Ph.D. is Professor of Film Studies and Rhetoric at the University of California, Berkeley and teaches about popular moving-image genres, modes, and media embodiment. Her books include: *Hard Core: Power, Pleasure and the Frenzy of the Visible* and *Playing the Race Card: Melodramas of Black and White, from Uncle Tom to O.J. Simpson*. She is currently completing a book entitled *Screening Sex*.

Yolanda Wimberly, M.D., M.Sc. is an Assistant Professor of Clinical Pediatrics at Morehouse School of Medicine in Atlanta, Georgia who practices adolescent medicine and is on staff at Grady Health Systems in Atlanta and at Clark Atlanta University Student Health Center.

Brandee Woleslagle is a Master's degree candidate at San Francisco State University in the Human Sexuality Studies Program.

Acknowledgments

The editors would like to sincerely thank Joyce Nishioka, Editorial Assistant, and Ruslan Valeev, Administrative Manager, for their tireless and careful work coordinating this project and contributing valuable perspectives from the outset. We also want to thank each of the authors whose academic and advocacy work has made this collection possible. This book has also been enriched by the keen editorial support we have received at Routledge, and we extend our appreciation to our Editor, Grace McInnes, and the editorial team headed by Sue Leaper at Florence Production. Finally, we wish to thank the Ford Foundation for its generous support of the National Sexuality Resource Center and the American Sexuality magazine project.

Introduction

Gilbert Herdt and Cymene Howe

In the twenty-first century, sexuality has become more public than ever before—with the media and Internet serving as new vehicles for sexual expression. This anthology explores how these changes in sexuality have influenced American culture and in turn have been influenced by the global society. Today, sexuality is more present in print media, television and film, but it is also more talked about than it has been in the past. Yet the real revolution in sexuality is how the Internet has infused our thinking, intimate relations, and politics. For the first time in history people are making friends and finding sexual and romantic partners online, some of which result in marriages and long-term relationships. People are also forging political movements online as never before. These transformations in intimacy and politics have expanded the ways that we think about sexuality, too. Such changes in technology and social development and political change also go a long way in explaining why sexuality has taken on an unprecedented importance in the twenty-first century.

This book serves two kinds of purpose. It provides an overview of many of the contemporary dynamics, including politics, regarding sexuality in the United States and around the globe in the twenty-first century—often from an "insider's" point of view. Additionally, the chapters are analytically challenging, providing new ways to think about sexuality, in all of its meanings, in many cultural contexts, online, and in the "real world."

The definition of sexuality has expanded dramatically in the past generation. It has come to mean not simply sex, but gender identities and roles, sexual orientation, eroticism, pleasure, intimacy, and reproduction, all of which correspond to the way that Americans have come to understand sexuality today.[1] The Web[2] is an enormous and expanding global information platform, providing new forms of communication as well as new romantic and sexual possibilities for individuals and groups. The Internet helps people to become sexually literate by facilitating sexual experiences that allow people to create new identities and sexual communities. These tools also support political advocacy for new sexual rights and social justice in the US and globally. This anthology provides rich but succinct materials through which the student can make a study of such changes online and in real social encounters.

Tracking the changing faces of sexuality and encouraging new kinds of sexuality education, is part of the mission of a major online magazine, *American Sexuality* (americansexuality.org).[3] *American Sexuality* features the work of interdisciplinary research scholars, social scientists, advocates, and teachers in the fields of anthropology, sociology, psychology, and health—striving to better understand sexuality in the context of US and global cultures. This book draws together many of the stories and experiences of diverse individuals and groups, as well as cutting-edge research in the field of sexuality studies that we have gathered through our work with *American Sexuality*. We particularly support the positive side of sexuality, while also providing the information needed to separate fact from fiction and science from superstition.

"Sexuality + Internet" brings revolutionary change. Both the cultural and individual meanings surrounding sexuality have undergone such a radical transformation that sexuality will never be the same again. From our vantage point, communications technologies and the community platforms they provide constitute a new "digital sexual revolution" shaping the way people understand, experience, and live their sexuality in the twenty-first century. Using the Internet as a powerful tool to address structural inequalities between sexual cultures, young people and social scientists, alike, have engaged a new way of thinking about the nature of sexual inequalities in the world today (Teunis and Herdt, 2006). This book is about the many sides of contemporary sexuality and gender in the real world and on the Internet—both of which suggest that we are in a new era for sexuality and for sexuality studies.

Surprisingly, this new sexual revolution has not been a part of school curricula or integrated into most classrooms. Quite a few universities now offer courses on sexuality and the Internet,[4] but as of yet, few of these general courses on gender, sexuality, women, and lesbian, gay, bisexual, transgender, and queer (LGBTQ) identities have incorporated the world of online sexuality into their curricula. Sexuality online is, broadly understood, an array of informational websites and recreational services related to romance and dating, sexual health, and diverse sexual and gender communities on the Internet. Information about sexuality now comes via digital books, research papers about sexuality and sexual development, and ever multiplying media sources from TV, newspapers, and magazines to blogs, MySpace, and Facebook.

Increasingly, the media portrays sexuality online as a preoccupation of young people, with some spending up to fifteen hours a day on the Internet, much of it devoted to friendship, sexual and romantic interests, and games. Undoubtedly some of this content online concerns parents, who may already face difficulties addressing sexual development in their children. Meanwhile, the commercialization of the Internet has accelerated at a dizzying pace: providing packaged sex and literally millions of commercial sites, selling products from Viagra to pornography and sex toys. Not long ago a *New York Times* article about a new strain of HIV reported that many men now use the Internet for finding sexual partners, bypassing bars and other social spaces. As authors such as Yorghos Apostologpoulous *et al.* point out in this book, the incidence of HIV infection is often predicated, not simply on individual risk behaviors, but upon the larger social contexts in which people make choices about their sexual health. Dating and sexual services are becoming more frequent on the Internet, and with this has come a rise in incidents of exploitation and victimization. In very public spaces, such as shopping malls and high schools, young people now also use cell phones to text message for dates, seeking out romantic and sexual relationships. Parents and the older generation remain relatively oblivious to these changes in how dating and relationships are being shaped by technology in this new information age.

Exploring sexuality via new technologies poses many challenges to people—how do you separate the good from the bad, the ludicrous from the dangerous, or truth from fiction? How do you make decisions about online dating, sexual health, pornography, and romantic experiences, and how do you avoid sexual predation? Teachers, understandably, may be hesitant to introduce these topics into discussion. However, these experiences are already happening right there in the classroom, through cell phones, laptops, handhelds, iPods, and other bridging technologies that connect people. In order to better understand the cultural changes we are all facing, we need to think broadly and comprehensively.

This collection addresses the sweeping changes that are unfolding before us everyday. *21st Century Sexualities* is divided into five parts. We begin with "Sexual Literacy and Learning Sexuality" seeing sexuality, not merely as a biological process or "drive," but as something that is learned and socially constructed. In "www., TV, and Sexual Commodification" we query how technologies, the media, and sexuality as a commodity are changing how we negotiate our sexuality on a daily basis. In the third part of this collection, "Sexual Health, Wellness and Medical Models," the medicalization of sexuality is critiqued. Here, we also recognize the dire need for medically accurate and easily (and anonymously) accessible information on sexually transmitted infections (STIs) and unintended pregnancies. As Yolonda Wimberly and Sandra Moore point out, honest communication with physicians is critical particularly considering the health disparities faced by many communities of color in the United States. The articles collected in "Sexual Activism and Rights" and "The Globalization of Sexuality" —such as Joyce Nishioka's discussion of the Cesar Chavez Institute and Cymene Howe's article on sexuality activism in Nicaragua—identify strategies and new models of activism in the United States and transnationally.

Sexual literacy and twenty-first century sexuality

Today's world requires a new kind of pedagogy that teaches people how to navigate sexuality online and make use of a vast new world of informational tools and data, while also sorting fact from fantasy. In this book we call that goal sexual literacy. Sexual literacy is defined here, and in Gilbert Herdt's chapter, as the ways in which people become knowledgeable and healthier sexual beings—protecting themselves from HIV/AIDS and STIs, avoiding unintended pregnancy, and understanding sexual violence such as date rape. Indeed, as both Ann Cahill and Leslie Simon describe in their respective articles on rape, understanding the meaning of rape in society is critical to eliminating it. One of our goals in supporting "sexual literacy" is to follow the US Surgeon General's lead in helping young people make healthy sexual choices.[5] The United States has fallen behind other Western countries in creating healthy sexual communities because it has not followed the advice of the top medical doctor in the United States. Part of the reason has to do with the way that politics and ideology have replaced science and education.[6] But sexual literacy also centers on the positive side of sexuality—learning to enjoy and appreciate sexual identities, the body, romance, pleasure, and intimate relations. The process of becoming sexually literate links individuals to larger communities and ultimately to society, supporting individual development and democracy.

People in their teens and twenties have grown up with the Internet. It is not surprising that many students think in ways adapted to this new technology. For young people today, information has always been just a few clicks away. But sometimes the information is biased, inaccurate, or saturated with politics. Young people think differently about the world because they are able to communicate with friends from across the country or across the globe. And yet, there are many differences in education, cultural models, and values surrounding sexuality. So far, this developmental experience with the Internet has hardly been reflected in what or how college students learn in the classroom. Meanwhile, as this technological revolution has occurred, sex education in schools and in the public domain has gone on the defensive. The US government's official policy promoting "abstinence only" sex education undermines sexual literacy (as Cynthia Rothschild shows in "Abstinence Goes Global: The United States, the Right Wing, and Human Rights").

The new ease and comfort of working with computers and on the Internet creates a distinct developmental subjectivity—or way of thinking about sexuality—that makes sexuality online seem normal and natural. Yet this is all so new! Sexuality and the Internet intersect, but there are also more familiar domains of learning about sexuality through experiences in school, like the "myths" we hear growing up, as Mariamne H. Whatley describes in "Folklore and the Sexual Lives of Adolescents." The media poses developmental challenges for young Black men—as Linwood J. Lewis describes in "Contesting the Dangerous Sexuality of Black Male Youth"—which coincides with the experience of many people of color who face racism and discrimination. On the other hand, Judith Halberstam finds children's media, like the movie *Finding Nemo*, reflecting potentially transgressive narratives that allow for more gender and sexual ambiguity than one might expect from Hollywood fare. Living with the Internet over the past decade, young people have forged a revolution without fully realizing its implications.

Sexuality and reproductive research: just now catching up with the digital sexual revolution

Given the huge changes introduced by the digital revolution at the advent of the twenty-first century, it should not be surprising that sexual cultures have adopted this new electronic platform. However, few experts predicted it. As recently as the mid 1990s, experts reviewing sexuality research and policy completely ignored the Internet.[7] The Web, meanwhile, grew exponentially. When President Clinton came into office in 1992, for example, there were fewer than a hundred websites and email correspondence was uncommon. Fourteen years later, as many as seven million new sites are added to the World Wide Web daily, some 50 to 80 percent originating in the United States alone (Schrader, 2002). There are literally tens of millions of websites, blogs, chat rooms, and online commercial venues associated with cybersex and sexual and romantic interactions online. In other words, sexuality has been a critical element in motivating the emergence of the Internet and the new cultural forms we find online. A new world of sexual identity formation, sexual health information, and sexual rights advocacy and debate has been born in this medium.

Sex has expanded exponentially on educational, commercial, governmental, political, and personal websites and blogs. However, the study of sexuality and reproductive health has fallen far behind this massive increase in sexual information online. In many of these venues, sexuality is portrayed as an individual issue, as something medical, or, in the words of Leonore Tiefer in this collection, "medicalized." WebMD and a variety of related sites provide excellent sexual health information. But it is important to recognize that sexuality is also a social, cultural, political, and legal issue, subject to definition by the government at times and often the topic of debates. As Stanton E. Samenow describes, a fixation on medical reasoning in the case of "sex addiction" can too easily dismiss abusive behavior. Legal dictates that define certain behaviors, identities, and relationships as "good" and integral to "good citizenship" are part and parcel of defining putatively "appropriate" persons in the contemporary United States. Often, these political and legal codes are extended to include what is acceptable in schools, neighborhoods, towns, and communities, as Jessica Fields and Celeste Hirschman describe in their article. The "culture wars" (Duggan and Hunter, 1995) that have raged over issues such as abstinence-only education, abortion rights, and same-sex marriage exemplify the volatile debates that erupt when culture, society, and sexuality are brought together in public forums.

The lag in how sexuality education is taught is another important reason for the gap between sexuality, reproductive research and the digital sexual revolution. Sex education, as it is bandied about in the culture wars, Janice Irvine (2002) notes, is largely confined to classrooms, school boards, and community meetings. It is notable that the major battles over abstinence-only sex education, the official US government policy, center entirely on the classroom, not on the Internet, even though new technologies of sexual information are clearly having an enormous impact on what we know and learn about sexuality. In short, the major institutions of our society, especially public education in middle and high schools, have failed to keep up with the technological revolution in the arenas of sexuality education, health, and rights. In fact, there are powerful contradictory trends online. As Deborah Levine suggests here, the Web has expanded what is considered "normal" sexuality, even as certain extremist groups aim to restrict what counts as normal in the definition of sexuality.

Today, in our late capitalist market economy, we should not be surprised to find that money and power are inextricably linked to sexuality and romance online. Sex and adult entertainment is big business. Billions of dollars are spent on commercial online venues, including those devoted to hardcore pornography. Some of America's most prestigious media companies net billions of dollars of annual profit from these adult entertainment platforms, while very little money is spent to promote sexual literacy. Obviously, the market for sexual entertainment is strong, provoking moral and political concerns for many people. It is important that sexual education not fall by the wayside. As any perusal of the Internet will show, many websites use sexual imagery or content and spam with gratuitous and often offensive sexual content, even when there is no apparent connection to the stated goals of the Web host. Despite the exponential growth of sexual content online, many people still fail to appreciate how easily sexual cultures have adapted to the Internet. How did American sexuality get to such a place? A brief glance at its history over recent decades sheds light on this question.

A history of sexuality: from moral panic to moral panic

The sexual history of the United States follows from important social, economic, racial, and political fault lines that have been intensively studied.[8] A brief history of sexuality after World War II shows how the rise of the Web is a dramatic departure from the past. America has a legacy of sexuality that reveals repeated cycles of "sexual hygiene," "social purity" movements, and crises in gender politics. Sexuality in America has been subject to "moral panics"—that is, periods when sexuality becomes a heightened political, moral, or ideological issue. Rather than focusing upon intimacy, romance, and sound public health, these periods of panic place attention on questions of morality that are, not surprisingly, contentious, embattled, and often cyclical. Coined in the early 1970s by British sociologist Stanley Cohen to identify "conditions, persons, episodes, and groups that are defined as a threat to societal values and interests," moral sexual panics have historically inflamed such issues as masturbation, abortion and reproductive rights, teen pregnancy, homosexuality, AIDS, and, most recently, marriage rights for gay and lesbian people.

A notable review of the field of sexuality research conducted by sociologist John Gagnon and anthropologist Richard Parker in 1995 identified several fundamental transformations that have occurred during this turbulent period of history. A key change they uncovered was a shift in epistemologies, or ways of knowing. In researching sexuality, some scholars moved away from psychoanalytic frameworks and began to favor social and cultural approaches to understanding sexual processes. Methodologies also changed among some researchers, from clinical or psychological survey methods to more social and cultural approaches. With these shifts in scientific thinking, there was an expansion in the populations studied, including homosexuals, women, and diverse ethnic and racial communities. Finally, researchers realized the key importance of the media, following the tremendous attention paid to the famed studies of zoologist Alfred Kinsey beginning in 1948. As dramatized in the film *Kinsey*, Kinsey's work got him on the cover of *Time* magazine and awakened America to the chasm between small town ideals of sexuality (which excluded masturbation and extramarital sexual relations) and the realities of Americans' sexual behavior.

Government-funded studies in the late 1950s to 1970s tended to focus on adolescent mothers and unintended pregnancy. Following the invention of the birth control pill in 1964, a greater "de-coupling" of reproduction and sexual behavior began to occur in American attitudes toward sexuality. The work of psychologists Masters and Johnson dramatically demonstrated a shift in understanding: sexuality was not only a matter of reproduction, but also one of pleasure and intimacy. In particular, women's sexuality became an important new arena through which to understand the complexity of human sexuality. During the 1960s, the "sexual revolution" saw the advent of what Edward Laumann and colleagues (1994) referred to as "recreational sex" in American culture. Gradually displacing an older discourse on disease, sexual dysfunction, and gender abnormalities, was a newer dialogue about adult consensual pleasure and intimacy. Social constructionist views on sexuality have rightly emerged and are gradually replacing the "disease model" that has so often pathologized female sexuality. However, as Leonore Tiefer describes in this collection, this has not meant the end of medicalizing sexuality. Meanwhile, new forms of sexual citizenship—that is, the full acceptance of sexual identities within public life—have became a part of society, media, and individual development (Weeks, 1985). Years later sexual citizenship remains highly contested, as it is in the question of whether same-sex couples have the right to marry or adopt children.

Feminism and gay and lesbian rights movements further shifted American sexuality. The women's health movement in the 1970s created a new paradigm for women taking charge of their health. Following the landmark decision of *Row* v. *Wade* in 1973, abortion rights were established and back-alley abortions and coat-hanger surgeries were laid to rest. Coincidentally, in that same year, the American Psychiatric Association declassified homosexuality as a disease, beginning a transformation in debates about sexual rights and the lives of LGBT people in the United States.

Beginning in the late 1970s and early 1980s, sexuality education became increasingly embattled and the focus of a new wave of sexual conservatives. This political transformation grew during the emergence of the AIDS epidemic in the early 1980s when homosexuals, commercial sex workers, Haitian immigrants, and others were targeted as scapegoats. This rising tide of reaction led to moral panic surrounding homosexuality but, paradoxically, it provided unprecedented funding for research on gay men, lesbians, bisexuals, and their communities since HIV prevention became an urgent public health priority. Bisexuality also came to be viewed as a "bridge" to HIV and STI infection (Gagnon, 2004). The twin concepts of "desire" and "danger" became central new vantage points for sexuality research and education during this time (Vance, 1984) and have continued to be influential, now, increasingly, on television and online. As Kathy Sisson points out here in her discussion about S/M activism, online communities provide new ways of talking about desire and danger, providing fertile territory for exploring new variations in sexual and emotional relationships among heterosexuals.

Compared to other "First World" or "developed" countries, the United States continues to have an abysmal level of sexual literacy. The continued prevalence of HIV transmission, unintended pregnancies, sexual violence, STIs, abortion complications, and homophobic violence in US high schools, as Christine Pettett describes in "Homophobia and Harassment in School-Age Populations," all point toward a decline in sexual literacy. The *quantity* of research on sexuality has generally been on the increase but the relative rise in sexual literacy has been low. The sheer increase in sexuality information should have resulted in a well-educated public but because of cultural and political forces has remained largely unrealized.

The 1990s opened new paradigms concerning sexual rights among research scholars, influenced by sexual health and rights advocacy, LGBT social movements, and emphases on gender and feminist perspectives (Parker *et al.*, 2000). Sexuality became increasingly politicized and fiscally conservative—an integral element of what Lisa Duggan and others have described as the neoconservative social, political, and sexual movement (2003). Masturbation, for example, became a topic of scientific study and public health discussion; yet Dr Jocelyn Elders, MD, was immediately fired from her position as US surgeon general for just mentioning that masturbation might provide an alternative to risky sexual practices (Irvine, 2005). Growing partly from the AIDS-prevention and education movement, queer politics and advocacy also emerged as a challenge to liberal articulations of gay and lesbian identity (Vaid, 1995; Warner, 1999; Howe, 2001). Intellectual innovations intent on "queering" the social sciences and humanities (Foucault, 1978; Butler, 1990) were also instrumental in rethinking transgender identity and practice. While gender nonconformity, akin to contemporary transgender sensibilities, certainly existed in the United States prior to this time (Kennedy and Davis, 1993; Feinberg, 1993), the 1990s saw new opportunities for creating transgender communities. Now, as Jillian Weiss explains in this collection, transgender people are challenging their workplaces to adequately provide for gender diversity. Only near the close of the twentieth century has an online transgender movement emerged, capitalizing on the Internet as a unique platform for mobilizing a global transgender movement—one of the most dramatic forms of new social justice advocacy using the Web (Herdt, 2004). Perhaps because there are few "symbolic homes" for transgender people in society, online venues have become extremely important. As Rita M. Melendez suggests in her article, many transgender people are vulnerable to discrimination and HIV infection; at the same time, Jamison Green points out that new opportunities for transforming one's gender have become more accessible and acceptable in recent years.

The pedagogy of sexuality has radically changed with the introduction of online materials. The coupling of the digital revolution with the pioneering Surgeon General's report (*Call to Action*) on comprehensive sexuality education in the US (Satcher, 2001) represents a watershed of change. Notably, this is the only Surgeon General's Report, one which covered topics such as the health risk of smoking, that was never officially endorsed by the US Government. The Report was released to provide a counterweight to the US government's official policy on "Abstinence Only" education rather than the previously widely used "comprehensive sexuality education" policy (which included education on abstinence and use of contraceptives, etc.). Abstinence-only is an educational policy largely bereft of scientific credibility (Kirby, 1997). To understand these federal policies, as Martha Kempner points out here, we must acknowledge the contemporaneous rise of the abstinence-only-until-marriage movement. The US government opposed publication of the Report and it was bitterly contested by right-wing anti-sex education organizations (Irvine, 2002). The emphasis on abstinence-only, as Renée T. White and Cynthia Pope describe in "Global Impact: US Sexual Health and Reproductive Policy," has not been limited to the United States but also has had global impact since these policies are deployed worldwide.

In the 1990s, sexual rights as a human right became established. Sexual rights, a concept growing from "women's rights as human rights" and the United Nation's conferences and forums on the status of women, have proliferated in many places around the world. As Sonia Corrêa notes in "Global Perspectives on Sexual Rights," the concept of universal human rights has changed the way governments and international governmental networks, such as the United Nations, now treat sexuality. Adrienne Germain and Jennifer Kidwell explain, for example, how the "feminization of AIDS" is a phenomenon that must be addressed at the international level. Just as the second wave of feminism and gay and lesbian rights movements from the 1960s and 1970s in the United States changed the shape of society and research on sexuality, so too do sexual rights discourses now impact the way in which rights on the global stage are advocated. Admittedly, however, sexual rights remain challenging to American society.

Sexuality in the twenty-first century has been changed by online sexuality, sexual politics, and emerging sexual cultures that have come through a variety of national and international debates, both old and new. From abstinence-only policies in school sex education, medicalization and sexual dysfunction in popular culture, abortion and reproductive politics, same-sex marriage debates, the "Don't Ask, Don't Tell Policy" in the military, and the media's role in representing all these dynamics—we have found that in order to successfully engage with the study of education, health, rights, and culture in general, one must first understand how these sexual controversies are linked to broader concerns in science and research. Our approach incorporates the theoretical and substantive perspectives of gender and socioeconomic status, race and ethnicity, sexual diversity, and disability. We also know that advocates are looking for a "big picture." In order to undertake productive activist work, one needs to know how these issues fit together with theory and politics as part of a larger cultural system. In light of the historical changes we have experienced in the United States around sexuality, what meanings are now attributed to sexuality, broadly, in our culture?

Searching: making meaning out of sexuality online

Reviewing history provides a context for thinking about changes in sexuality theory, methodology, and themes in both American society and research priorities. While expanding meanings and practices of sexuality, romance, and intimacy online may have seemed inevitable, as we have shown, they are so recent that rules and norms have not yet been established to fully deal with these changes. Based on these dramatic shifts, we have found key themes that frame how we understand sexual desire, sexual politics, gender and sexual behavior, HIV/STIs, and adolescent and adult sexual behavior and intimate relations:

- The *pedagogy of sexuality* is sex education online, gender and reproductive information, and, to a lesser extent, sexual rights. But it is more than that, too. As we spend more time online and begin to form social spaces and sexual lives there, we now face fundamental shifts in the way we understand sexuality.
- *Sexual health and wellness* constitutes a sea of information online—some specious and some accurate—about sexual health, behavior, transmission, and treatment. This wealth of information is often politicized, requiring a careful analysis of the *sources* of information.
- The *Internet, online worlds, and the commodification of sexual experience* are all issues we have to deal with today. Think of online dating, blogs and chat rooms, adult entertainment and pornography, online commercial sex websites, and the multiple sites available to create intimate relationships, often organized for profit.
- *New sexual communities* have formed online and in the "real world." These are now often the spaces where identities are formed, advocacy strategies planned, and communities created—transgender and intersex communities being recent and important case in point.
- The Internet has also led the way to *global interconnections, communications, and political and social justice advocacy*. It is no secret that the Internet has shaped media and advocacy strategies. From local nonprofits to global organizations such as the United Nations or Amnesty International, online advocacy now crosses many borders. For sexual rights, the online world is now a key staging ground for innovations in social justice struggles, where ideas and political practices from multiple cultures and political contexts can be exchanged.

The tremendous availability of sexuality online can have the negative effect of reproducing racial and heterosexist stereotypes about gender, sexual, and ethnic minorities in particular. These stereotypes, like the sexual panic surrounding the "down low" in African American communities, existed long before the Internet. But they have been exaggerated by television, print media, and the Web, as Gilberto R. Gerald points out here. The media may perpetuate "bi-phobia" or erasure, as Loraine Hutchins writes. Or, as Gregory Rebchook and Alberto Curotto point out, Internet chatrooms may reinforce stereotypes about gay men being "overly" interested in sexual encounters. The Internet also provides a new space of pedagogy for queer, transgender, and straight youth who find support in their efforts to mobilize responses to homophobia in the schools. As these advocacy perspectives show, the Internet allows a means of avoiding intolerance, hostility, and judgment online and expanding the concept of what is "normal."

But how far can normality extend, some authors ask? For example, can a man with cerebral palsy or spinal cord injury actually "do that"—that is, engage in sex? Russell P. Shuttleworth notes in "Disability and Sexuality: From Medical Model to Sexual

Rights" that people often ask this question, following the stereotype that people with disabilities do not have a sexual life. From Shuttleworth's vantage point, disability rights must be about more than access to buildings and employment; they must include sexual rights for disabled persons. Tre Trefethen would agree: since he became wheel-chair bound, dating, sex, and love are perhaps more important to him now than before his accident. In these and others cases, as Gloria González-López describes, a fundamental question for minority populations in teaching and learning about sexuality is: How do we challenge inequalities?

As we consider how we now negotiate sexuality online and in our lives, it may be helpful to remember an important theory introduced by sociologist John Gagnon (2004)—the sexual script. Scripts are the means by which sexual interactions are socially organized, according to Gagnon, providing "lines" and "roles" for people to play as if they were performers on stage. Sexual scripts help provide the necessary beliefs and meanings to accompany each stage of sexual development as well as the changes that occur from one life stage to the next, from childhood to young adulthood for example. Sexual scripts have three primary dimensions: *intrapsychic*, what goes on inside someone's head; *interpersonal*, guides to intimate relations in dating, courtship, marriage, extramarital relations, etc.; and *cultural*, the specific and often gender-specific rules and beliefs for playing out a role in a particular sexual culture, institution, and social event.

The Internet, it should be fairly obvious, blurs the boundaries between these different types of sexual scripts. Take for example online gaming, which involves hundreds of thousands of individuals. As Brandee Woleslagle reports from her research about *Everquest*, some people locate romantic partners and even find marriage through their personas online. When someone's private reality can be merged with their online world, and then collectively transformed through an online game, chat room, or symbolic identity, the personal and the cultural become reflected and connected as never before.

Sexual roles, identities, and activities in the online medium are highly ambiguous, allowing for the creation of new sexual networks. Television commercials that promote dating services are indirectly driving people to these new electronic venues for romance, love, and sexual connection. Television, film, and commercial pornography also tend to blur the sexual scripts that have existed in US culture. TV shows such as *Will and Grace* and *The L Word* have made great strides toward expanding viewers' sense of sexual diversity, working to "normalize" gay and lesbian identities and practices. However, as Kris Scott Martí notes here about *The L Word*, critiques can be leveled about the commodification of lesbian and gay identities. In cable TV shows such as *Six Feet Under,* subjects, such as abortion, are brought into the public domain through entertainment, but not without controversy, as Tracy Weitz and Anthony Hunter note in their review.

In the world of online relationships and TV portrayals, readers may ask: Isn't this just an illusion, imagination, or fantasy? Perhaps television, media, and pornography do appear this way with their mass appeal and high profit dimensions. Are we witnessing a phenomenon that is "onscence" rather than one that is "obscene"? asks Film Studies and Rhetoric scholar Linda Williams. The porn industry produces immense quantities of material designed for sexual entertainment, and as Amy Sueyoshi describes, some of this material reproduces racial and gender stereotypes. Cutting across the world of televised and online images is the commodification of sexuality. In some sense, this is nothing new: we have all heard the hackneyed expression that "prostitution is the world's oldest profession." But with the rapid circulation of images and the trafficking of people, rights regarding sex work and pressing questions about transnational sex work are critical matters of our times. Juhu Thukral describes how combating sexual trafficking has become central to activists working on both local and global levels, though often to the exclusion of other social justice concerns. The advent of sex work on a global scale has been augmented by the Internet, though again, it certainly preceded the Internet. While Katherine Frank analyzes the motives of men for visiting strip clubs and its socioeconomic dimensions, Ann M. Lucas underscores the racialized and gendered dimensions of sex work on the streets of the United States. Jakob Rigi and Christophe Robert provide international dimensions of changing values around sex work, respectively on "moral economies" in Russia and "foreign plague" discourses in Vietnam.

Of course, sexual health, risk, and wellness are not fantasies—they are real and can have deadly consequences if mishandled or handled with ignorance. A decision made in the heat of passion, conditioned by social values or motivated by love, can have lifelong health effects. Whether for women seeking abortion care in rural settings, as described by Carole Joffe in "Bringing Medical Abortion to Rural America: Interview with an Abortion Provider" or among aging men and women across the country who are at risk for HIV infection, as described by David M. Latini and David W. Coon, concerns that appear to center on private decisions are in fact couched in very public policies generally. Medicine, itself, for Angel Foster *et al.*, has now become a site for health advocacy among some medical students, who are trying to change the politics of the medical industry. In rural settings too, as Cathleen Willging and colleagues show, homophobia impacts the provision of mental healthcare for indigenous people and Latino/as in the southwestern United States. Medicine and healthcare are not areas without controversy, which is especially clear in debates around intersexuality and genital surgery. As David Cameron illustrates, these medical interventions have now become a concern of human rights activists. In all of these examples, the intersection of sexuality and medicine now often speaks to much broader arenas for social concern and activism.

Movements are afoot in the United States and other parts of the world to legalize marriage for gay men and lesbians. It is a unique moment in history that is controversial, strongly opposed by some and welcomed by others. Here, Robert M. Kertzner has reviewed these issues and provides a foundation for thinking about this latest chapter in the long history of the sexual rights movement. While same-sex marriage is controversial on the national political stage, the "normalization" of gay and lesbian relationships has also been contentious among some queer rights activists who aim to disrupt categories of sexuality and gender, and the trappings of marriage. Following Michael Warner's argument in *The Trouble With Normal*, has "normalcy" in gay and lesbian life been purchased to accommodate heterosexual norms at the expense of creating queer alternatives to social life?

Sexual rights movements and advocacy around the world have become one of the most fertile arenas for understanding sexuality. How are women able to negotiate condom use and remain healthy when their sexual and reproductive rights are questioned or undermined? Raising the rights of women following the Beijing Accord, trying to combat homophobia, or advocating for the rights of sexually trafficked persons are new arenas for thinking about social justice and offer new venues for mobilizing opposition to inequality. For example, the first official act of President George W. Bush was to re-instate the global "gag rule," which forbids US foreign aid funding to be given to family planning NGOs (non-governmental organizations) that provide counseling or referral for abortion, or which advocate to make abortion legal or more accessible in their countries (Girard, 2004). Abstinence-oriented HIV/AIDS prevention programs raise a new specter of US sexual and health policy influence abroad. In sexual and reproductive rights work, people are now questioning and critiquing the potential damage that has been done to women, men, and children's health in developing countries through such global programs.

The role of war, militaries, and peacekeepers are things not often associated with sexuality. However, it is very clear, especially in recent years, that these are deeply interrelated. Too often in the twentieth century, as Gilbert Herdt explains, hyper-masculinity, sexual humiliation, and rape are used as tools of war. As we enter new conflicts in the twenty-first century, such as the Iraq war, a fundamental question remains: Why does sexual conquest and sexual humiliation continue to be a part of war today? Genevieve Ames, Andrew Bickford, and Ann Russ show how military cultures become partially shaped by alcohol consumption and the intermediate social space of having a "leave" for recreational sex. Paul Higate, writing about the war-ravaged Congo, explains that condom distribution and notions of appropriate behavior and relationships with local people is critical for UN peacekeepers in the region. Sealing Cheng also describes the intimate relationship between militarization, US military bases in the Philippines, and the rise of sex work in and around these outposts. Does the relationship between war and sexual abuse reveal a dark side of human nature that requires further study? We suspect so. Connecting research to these real world challenges is a critical aspect of sexuality and gender studies today.

Sexual cultures and online sexual communities are not simply about finding sex, romance, and chat. They are, rather, sites that are filled with possibilities for cultural creativity, political change, and the emergence of new forms of human development and human rights. "Sex" or "sexuality" in our twenty-first century model, profoundly impacted by visual and communications media, does not preclude marriage and reproduction. Far from it. But neither does it imply a singular focus on love and marriage between men and women, as was typical in an earlier era of history. Today the Internet is transforming all these sexualities—and we invite you to reflect deeply on how your life is changing too, as you enter the world of these readings about sexuality online.

Notes

1   The World Health Organization suggests this omnibus working definition as well.
2   The Web is "made of many sites linked together; users can travel from one site to another by clicking on hyperlinks." Or "The World Wide Web is the universe of network-accessible information, an embodiment of human knowledge."—Tim Berners-Lee, inventor of the World Wide Web. Retrieved; On-line Encyclopedia, 1998.
3   A publication of the National Sexuality Resource Center at San Francisco State University— a long-term project supported by the Ford Foundation.
4   In 2000, The Program in Human Sexuality Studies at San Francisco State University created a regular elective course on Sexuality and the Internet, taught in a "smart classroom," that has been highly successful.
5   See *A Call to Action: Surgeon General David Satcher's Report* (2001) on sexual health, sexual health disparities, and the need for accurate information.
6   F. Girard (2004).

7   For example, in her 1995 (Ford Foundation funded) report on sexuality in the United States, Dr Diane DiMauro, one of the foremost leaders on sexuality and social issues in the US, did not need to mention the net in her comprehensive review of the scientific literature!

8   See, for example, J. Weeks, *Sexuality and Its Discontents* (New York: Routledge & Kegan Paul, 1985); J. D'Emilio and E. Freedman, *Intimate Matters* (New York: Harper & Row, 1988); and contrast Smith-Rosenberg, C. 1975. "The female world of love and ritual: Relations between women in nineteenth century America." *Signs* 1: 1–29.

References

Butler, J. 1990. *Gender Trouble: Feminism and the Subversion of Identity*. New York: Routledge.

DiMauro, D. 1995. *Sexuality Research in the United States*. New York: Social Science Research Council.

Duggan, L. 2003. *The Twilight of Equality? Neoliberalism, Cultural Politics, and the Attack on Democracy*. Boston, MA: Beacon.

Duggan, Lisa, and Nan D. Hunter. 1995. *Sex Wars: Sexual Dissent and Political Culture*. New York: Routledge.

Feinberg, L. 1993. *Stone Butch Blues: A Novel*. Ithaca, NY: Firebrand.

Foucault, Michel. 1978. *The History of Sexuality: An Introduction*. New York: Vintage.

Gagnon, J.H. 2004. *An Interpretation of Desire*. Chicago, IL: University of Chicago Press.

Gagnon, J. H., and R. Parker. 1995. *Introduction: Conceiving Sexuality*. New York: Routledge.

Girard, F. 2004. Global implications of US domestic and international policy on sexuality. *IWGSSP Working Paper No. 1*. New York: Columbia University.

Herdt, G. 2004. "Sexual development, social oppression, and local culture." *Sexuality Research and Social Policy* 1: 1–24.

Howe, Cymene. 2003. Queer pilgrimage: the San Francisco homeland and identity tourism. In Lee D. Baker (ed.) *Life in America: Identity and Everyday Experiences*. Oxford: Blackwell, pp. 284–264.

Irvine, Janice. 2002. *Talk About Sex*. Berkeley, CA: University of California Press.

Irvine, Judith. 2005. *Harmful to Minors*. Preface by Jocelyn Elders. Minneapolis, MN: University of Minnesota Press.

Kennedy, E., and M.D. Davis. 1993. *Boots of Leather, Slippers of Gold: The History of a Lesbian Community*. New York: Routledge.

Kirby, D. 1997. No easy answers: research findings on programs to reduce teen pregnancy. Washington, DC: National Campaign to Prevent Teen Pregnancy.

Laumann, E.O., J.H Gagnon, R.T. Michael, and S. Michaels. 1994. *The Social Organization of Sexuality: Sexual Practices in the United States*. Chicago, IL: University of Chicago Press.

Parker, R., M.R. Barbosa, and P. Aggleton (eds) 2000. *Framing the Sexual Subject: The Politics of Gender and Power*. Berkeley, CA: University of California Press.

Satcher, D. 2001. *The Surgeon-General's Call to Action to Promote Sexual Health and Responsible Sexual Behavior*. July 9, 2001. Available from URL: http://www.surgeongeneral.gov/reports publications.html.

Schrader, A.M. 2002. *Technology and the Politics of Choice: Information Literacy, Critical Thinking, and Intellectual Freedom*. March 15, 2002. Available from URL: http://www.learning resources.ab.ca/Freedom.html.

Teunis, N., and G. Herdt (eds) 2006. *Sexual Inequalities and Social Justice*. Berkeley, CA: University of California Press.

Vaid, U. 1995. *Virtual Equality: The Mainstreaming of Gay and Lesbian Liberation*. New York: Anchor Books.

Vance, Carole. 1984. *Pleasure and Danger: Toward a Politics of Sexuality*. New York: HarperCollins.

Warner, M. 1999. *The Trouble with Normal: Politics, and the Ethics of Queer Life*. New York: Free Press.

Weeks, J. 1985. *Sexuality and Its Discontents; Meanings, Myths, and Modern Sexualities*. New York: Routledge.

Part 1

Sexual literacy and learning sexuality

The very idea of needing to "learn" sexuality may seem like nonsense. After all, aren't we all born with innate sexual drives, desires, and the biological capacity to reproduce—making us all naturally sexual beings? Don't we all have a sexual self that is a physical, psychological, and emotional part of who we are? Well, yes and no. Clearly, we do not learn our sexuality in the same way that we learn the multiplication table or the periodic chart. And it is true that science has shown us a variety of physiological, endo-crinological, and developmental factors that influence our physical sexuality and hence our sexual selves. But we also know that the cultural and social environments in which we grow up and live have at least as much, if not more, to do with how we think about, and live, our sexuality.

This Part is an opportunity to consider how it is that we each learn about sexuality—whether through personal experience, through friends and family, in school, or, increasingly, online. But even beyond considering how you have learned your sexuality as an individual, this Part asks you to think about how society and the cultural contexts in which we live actually shape and determine how we learn about sexuality and, ultimately, how we behave. Learning sexuality encompasses many processes over time—shaping how we think about our bodies, our desires, our emotions as well as how we relate to other people through those channels. Sexuality goes beyond our genitals to be sure. We now know that it involves the whole body. But sexuality is also profoundly influenced and learned according to the ways that our families, communities, and culture talk about, understand, and conceive of it. In this sense, our sexuality is not simply "ours" as individuals but part and parcel of larger social dynamics that are constantly unfolding around us.

From sex ed to sexuality education in schools

Many of us have had sex education classes. Sex ed in schools can be traced all the way back to the 1900s when a venereal disease epidemic in the United States led the Society of Sanitary and Moral Prophylaxis to insist that schools prepare young people to protect themselves from disease. For the next fifty years, schools and organizations—such as the YMCA and the National Education Association—created and taught sex education, not only to maintain public health, but also to promote gender roles and behaviors considered appropriate for males and females. Priority was placed on making positive choices through knowledge about one's body rather than on practicing avoidance techniques associated with earlier VD-prevention curricula.

In the 1980s sex education in schools also began to question traditional gender role socialization and included diversity components in the curricula, allowing non-heterosexual students to see themselves reflected in a range of human sexual behaviors and identities. During this time, sex education in many schools broadened its purpose—becoming "sexuality education" that addresses human sexual diversity as well as strategies for avoiding disease and pregnancy. This was also the era of a new public health crisis: HIV/AIDS. Sexuality education needed to approach the epidemic from many angles, including instruction on the proper use of condoms and strategies to build self-esteem in order to encourage less risky sexual behaviors. In some sense, sex ed had come full circle: from a concern with sexually transmitted diseases, to a stress on family planning and alternative sexualities, and back again to a focus on disease transmission. The 1980s were also the beginning of the battles around sex education, which continue into the present.

The big questions and controversies surrounding sex education have revolved around how much information young people should receive about contraception (birth control) and different kinds of sexual practices and sexual identities. For many, the question is: If young people hear about these things aren't they more likely to do them? For others, the real concern is about young people having access to a wide range of information so they can make good decisions about their sexual behavior and identities. As one would imagine, sexuality education curricula has led to charged controversies about the morals and values underlying each of these approaches. Heated debates around what should be included and what should be excluded continue to rage in school board meetings, church gatherings, and the national political arena. Currently, federal dollars are being funneled into "abstinence only until marriage" sex education curricula and teaching. This approach to educating young people has not been scientifically proven to delay intercourse, prevent pregnancy, or curb the spread of STDs, but its core tenet—namely that teens should not have sex until they are married—seems to appeal to many policymakers.

Understanding sexuality in context

To think that we learn about sex and sexuality only in school would be naive. Many of us talk with friends about sexual techniques and experience during adolescence and sometimes throughout our entire lives. Talking about sex and sexual feelings with friends is a great thing if you feel comfortable doing so. But, of course, there is always the question about whether the information you are getting is accurate. Can you get herpes if you use a condom? Is homosexuality a lifestyle choice or biologically determined from birth? Some answers can be found by going to good, reliable sources of sexual health information. Other questions are really better understood through talking, analyzing, and thinking about what sexuality means for you, your friends, family, and social world. In this Part, it will also become very clear that not everyone has an equal opportunity to learn about, explore, and think about their feelings around sexuality. There are ways that racial and gender stereotypes impact the way we see others, and sometimes ourselves. The media, for one, continues to play a major role in what we consider attractive, what we desire, and what we think is a "correct" kind of sexuality. This Part puts these kinds of questions up for discussion. Here you can challenge what you think you know about sexuality and consider learning through a new set of lenses.

1 What is sexual literacy, and why is it needed now?

Gilbert Herdt

Americans are fixated on sex. This obsession is age-old and not unique to the United States, but the packaging is new—and it is causing harm.

Contrary to what the pundits say, we do not love sex. We are deeply ambivalent about sexual pleasure and intimacy. Parents worry about whether their teens are "doing it." Teachers of sexuality education avoid mentioning the "P" word—that is, pleasure—because it inspires fear and near panic, even among parents. Why is this? Poor sexual literacy. Part of the problem is that sexuality education is too little and too late, and, for many people growing up, that leads to misunderstanding and fear. We can change the climate and this chapter suggests why we should.

Americans harbor a collective concern about issues such as unintended pregnancy, sexually transmitted diseases, and sexually active youth, and now fear, bordering on panic, of gays and lesbians gaining the right to marry. Indeed, moral panics are common in the history of American sexuality. The term "moral panics" was coined in the early 1970s by sociologist Stanley Cohen to identify conditions, persons, episodes, and groups that are defined as a "threat to societal values and interests." In the nineteenth century, the public viewed masturbation as a moral threat; in the twentieth century, people feared teen pregnancy, STDs, and abortion. Today's moral panics include homosexuality, HIV, and marriage equality. Unfortunately, sexuality is an easy target, and politicians have continuously employed a politics of moral panic to disrupt competent sexuality education. The tactic has succeeded to a degree because of sexual *illiteracy*, an inability to comfortably and competently discuss the many dimensions of sexuality. Sexual *literacy*, on the other hand, is the knowledge and skills needed to promote and protect sexual wellness—having healthy intimate relationships, being able to prevent disease, understanding sexuality beyond just the act of sex. Sexual wellness comes from having comprehensive sexuality education and then continuing to learn throughout life.

In contrast, our national fixation concerns sex that is packaged to market products or to titillate, rather than sexuality that is genuine, well rounded, and healthy. Commercial ad campaigns and other market forces, which are well planned and executed, produce and shape packaged sex. Packaged sex is the image of a curvaceous woman in lingerie plastered on a billboard, and television innuendos that sell everything from cars to cell phones. Packaged sex can be found in pornography, on reality TV shows, and even in the messages of extremist organizations opposed to sexuality education. Packaged sex is commercialized (sex for sale, sex for marketing). Packaged sex is also politicized (sex for votes), used to promote "morality" campaigns against sexuality education, abortion rights, and HIV prevention. Examined closely, these efforts to promote particular forms of sexuality, such as the movement for abstinence-only sex education, are grounded, not in ethics or scientifically based understanding, but rather in conventionalized morality that denies accurate knowledge to the young people who need it, and that marginalizes others.

As a nation, we fail to make progress with sexuality because we confuse packaged sex with genuine sexuality. Parents hesitate to have frank discussions about sexuality with their children, fearing the promotion of packaged sex and fearing that if they discuss the "P" word it will lead their offspring to become sexually promiscuous. While understandable, this fear is groundless. There is strong evidence to suggest that when young people get a good sex education they are much less vulnerable to sexual and gender abuse. Many educators are concerned about what happens when teens are *not* taught about ways to avoid pregnancy, sexually transmitted diseases, and date rape. In this packaged sex climate, however, many adults flinch from any mention of sex, either as parents at home or as teachers in the classroom, because of extremist attacks on comprehensive sexuality education.

It's no wonder. We have reached a milestone for sexual *ill*iteracy in the United States. During the 2004 presidential campaign packaged sex clouded politics and distorted debate on issues such as abortion rights, marriage equality, and abstinence-only education. Obscenity was also a political football: remember Janet Jackson's "wardrobe malfunction" during the Super Bowl halftime performance? Through these panics extremist organizations fanned the flames of ignorance and successfully promoted sexual illiteracy. Democracy suffers in such a climate.

As a country we must realize that people are suffering. Studies show that medical doctors are uncomfortable asking patients the most basic questions about sexual health, questions that may provide critical indicators of mental and physical problems. Other studies indicate that healthcare professionals have failed to help teenagers with questions about sexual development. And many physicians admit being uncomfortable asking patients, young or old, about sexual abuse or violence, even when they suspect it. Though some people would be comfortable talking to leaders in their faith communities about sexual development and intimate relationships, ministers, rabbis, and imams often lack the knowledge and language to communicate and counsel effectively on these matters, even when they have the motivation to do so.

Ironically, as Americans, we pride ourselves on our love of progress. But when it comes to sexuality, we are lagging behind. American rates of unintended pregnancy, abortion, sexual coercion, and HIV infection are the highest in the industrial world. Rape and sexual violence are all too common. And the sexuality of individuals who are disadvantaged or discriminated against, whether by race, gender, orientation, class, or ability, suffers even more as a result of the sexual illiteracy that governs the national dialogue. As a result of our history of imposing ideology and morality upon science and public health, sexual literacy is in decline in the United States. In the major arenas of sexual health (including unintended pregnancy, STD rates, HIV infection, complications from abortion, sexual violence, and assaults related to gender and sexual orientation), we trail our Western allies. As with other arenas of social democracy and education, our society will continue to suffer until literacy improves and everyone shares alike in positive sexual health.

We need to encourage greater tolerance for and acceptance of sexuality and sexual literacy in American society. It is important for each of us—citizens, parents, teachers, spiritual beings, and policy makers—to speak out in support of sexual literacy for all. Only then can we break the vicious cycle that has led to treating sex, not as something precious about the human condition, but as a package for sale or for the promotion of fear. Someone wise once commented that a journey of a thousand miles must begin with a single step. Take the step toward better sexual literacy today—read, go online, get better informed about sexuality to make a difference in the lives of those you care about!

2 Folklore and the sexual lives of adolescents

Mariamne H. Whatley

Whoever believes middle school students don't talk about sex without prompting from sexuality education classes is probably suffering from both amnesia and complete isolation from adolescents. Everyone surely remembers the sexual stories they heard as teens and preteens. As adults we may be shocked or amused by these stories, but we should not ignore them. Rather than dismissing a legend as ridiculous, impossible, or too disgusting, we should pay attention to adolescent legends and other folklore, such as beliefs and even jokes. By inviting adolescents to bring their folklore to family conversations or to the classroom, we may get a new perspective on their pressing concerns. By engaging with folklore and not dismissing it, we may have new avenues to approach adolescents' anxieties and fears.

Take this story, for example, told by a college student recalling middle school:

> When I was in seventh grade living in (hometown), there was a story about a girl (name). Supposedly she was experimenting in some solo sexual activity with a hot dog (that means masturbating with a hot dog, but of course no one said that word then; if they even said the word, usually you just got "the look") and it—the hot dog—got stuck. Her father had to take her to the emergency room. She went to one of the other junior highs in turn, so we never got a chance to stare at her and giggle, and I guess most of us forgot by the time we hit high school.

This story, which circulates in various forms through middle and high schools, is a contemporary legend, commonly known as an urban legend, and a form of folklore. Adolescents are a folk group—with many subgroups of jocks, cheerleaders, Goths, various racial and ethnic groups, LGBT (lesbian, gay, bisexual, and transgendered) students, and others. Folklore is the unofficial culture of a group, the means by which information and attitudes are transmitted and interpreted within the group. It is part of every individual's everyday life. Though folklore is often used as a synonym for false, it can be completely true in the sense of portraying actual events or being scientifically accurate. What is more important than folklore's accuracy is the truth folklore conveys about the attitudes, fears, and beliefs of a group, which in turn help shape and maintain the identity of the group.

We found in our research with young people that students repeatedly report stories similar to the hot dog legend. Does this mean that there is an epidemic of girls incompetently and disastrously experimenting with masturbation? Certainly not, but there are reasons why such stories are told again and again by adolescents and there is a lot that can be learned from them.

In these legends, masturbatory experiments by girls and young women result in humiliation at the very least, and sometimes escalate to emergency-room visits and even fatal infections. They demonstrate a lack of knowledge of anatomy and a strong discomfort with sexuality, particularly with the idea of women having sexual autonomy. Numerous legends show that girls' sexual desires and experimentation without a man merit severe folkloric punishment. These legends exert powerful social control over the girls who hear the stories: they learn what is not acceptable and they know who the "sluts" are, even if none of these alleged cases of masturbation actually occurred.

The girls in these legends are often not anonymous and in our research the women who told stories in their middle school years reported that students who did not fit in, who had physically developed early, or who were "weird" in some way were usually singled out. These stories can follow girls to high school and even college. Recent research about girls identified as sluts and the impact this labeling has had on them makes it clear how destructive such stories can be even beyond adolescence.

Spanish Fly, biology class, and social control

Fear of unleashing powerful sexual desire in young women appears in many folkloric forms. Moving beyond the naiveté of the hot dog experiments are such disturbing stories as this:

> This girl was out on a date and the guy gave her some Spanish Fly so that she'd be more receptive to his advances. He left her alone in the car for a few minutes and when he came back, he found she'd gotten so horny while he was gone that she'd impaled herself on the gear shift.

The legends often conclude that if the young woman survives such dramatic masturbation, "she had to change schools." The man who gave her the alleged aphrodisiac doesn't suffer and doesn't live under a cloud of rumor as does his victim. She is seen as sexually deviant; he as merely trying to make her "receptive."

Other stories, such as the following, demonstrate the role of folklore in social control:

> There is a story told in Augusta about a girl who attended a local high school. During sex ed class the subject of semen entered the discussion. During the discussion the teacher stated that semen was high in glucose. Suddenly the girl raised her hand and blurted out, "Then why does it taste so salty?" Realizing what she had done, she ran out of the room and transferred to a different high school the next day.

In other versions of this story, a biology teacher identifies sperm in a young woman's cheek scraping on a microscope slide. In these legends, the punishment for fellatio is not emergency surgery or death but total humiliation. Folklore can function as a warning about unacceptable behavior and what will happen if norms are violated.

Changing trends, changing stories

As social norms, technologies, and trends change, folklore shifts to accommodate social and cultural transformations. Recently, for example, we have begun to hear versions of these legends that substitute a young woman for a young man, with the telltale sperm serving to "out" him as gay to his entire class. Again, it doesn't matter if the stories are true; the message is still powerful and in this case helps to patrol the borders of heterosexuality.

A school counselor in the UK repeated a legend that had only recently begun to circulate. Numerous high school girls reported stories of other girls whose tongue-piercing got caught in a boy's foreskin during fellatio. These new legends get created because of the increased prevalence of both oral sex and body piercings in students' lives. As there is more pressure on young women to perform fellatio, there may come a time when humiliation in the classroom focuses on the young woman who does not know what semen tastes like.

Legends about HIV/AIDS have also changed in response to shifts in attitudes. For many years the predominant legend about HIV transmission was some version of the two tales below:

> There was this girl vacationing over spring break in Florida. She met some guy, and they fell in love. They did everything together and by the final night of vacation she conceded to sleeping with him. The next day as he saw her off, he gave her a small gift-wrapped box and told her not to open it until she got back to school. She got back, eagerly unwrapped it, and sat, numbly reading the inscription on the miniature coffin: "Welcome to the wonderful world of AIDS . . ."
> This guy went to Florida for spring break and he met this really beautiful lady in a bar. And they went back to his hotel room. When he woke up in the morning, she was gone but scrawled across the mirror in red lipstick was the message, "Welcome to the Wonderful World of AIDS."

Comparing these two chilling legends can give interesting insights into the stereotypes of what young women and men want in a sexual encounter—romance versus a one-night stand. They also conveyed very important messages about the risks of heterosexual sex at a time when that population felt protected. But these stories also reinforced the incorrect belief that it was strangers who carried HIV risk; adolescents explained their protection from HIV as "I only go out with people from my high school."

Legends about HIV transmission through heterosexual sex have been almost completely replaced by legends about hidden infected syringes that prick unsuspecting people watching a movie, pumping gas, or buying a can of soda. In one discussion with students, where I asked why they thought AIDS legends have changed, one student pointed out that it takes any blame away from someone who is HIV-positive because the emphasis is not on sexual transmission. "After all," she said, "everyone needs to buy a Coke." Of course, this new form of the folk legend also undermines messages about safer sex.

Other legendary dangers

There are other legends that give warnings to adolescents about sexual dangers they may face as they leave high school and go to college or other new settings. For example, young women are warned about the dangers of drinking and fraternities in a common and disturbing legend:

At a fraternity party, a girl drank too much and passed out leaning out the window. One of the fraternity brothers came into the room and saw her. He lifted up her dress and violated her. When he was done, he went and retrieved one of his friends from the party. He brought his friend into the room, and his friend violated the woman also. They decided to see who she was and so they pulled her in. They looked at her face and the second frat boy said, "Oh my God, that's my sister!"

While the women may learn to be wary of fraternity parties and heavy drinking, young men receive a message that may be read as, "Every woman is someone's sister, mother, daughter, so think (or at least look) before you rape."

These legends reflect a reality—an increased danger of sexual assault associated with alcohol consumption. Another common legend reflects imagined dangers from "predatory" gay men:

A student went to the doctor complaining of pain in his anus. The doctor claimed it was from anal intercourse, and the guy freaked out. He was not a homosexual and had never had anal intercourse, but the doctor said there was definitely evidence of this occurrence. Apparently his roommate was putting ether on his bed at night to knock him out and then proceeded to have anal intercourse with him. He had seen the ether and Vaseline in the room, but this was not unusual because the roommate was an entomology major. In the end, this roommate was kicked out of school.

These legends are troubling to hear, but if we pay attention to adolescent folklore, we have a better understanding of their fears, anxieties, and concerns. It also may give us ideas about what both formal and informal sexuality education should address. If students are talking about masturbation and oral sex, then educators, parents, and youth leaders ought to be ready to participate in the dialogue.

Talking about folklore

Adolescents talk to each other about a wide range of topics related to sexuality. In their folklore there is a lot of misinformation not just about scientific "facts" but also in terms of stereotyping, whether it is gay men, sexually active women, or fraternity brothers. Educators need to intervene in these conversations and move them into an environment where appropriate information can be provided and where values, ethics, and such topics as discrimination and violence can be explored. Folklore tells us what students are already thinking and talking about. Following the often rapidly evolving folklore can help us understand trends in adolescent sexual norms and attitudes.

The next time you hear a "gross," strange, or scientifically impossible story, don't dismiss it or its teller; listen to the messages behind the legend to learn what's really going on.

3   Contesting the dangerous sexuality of Black male youth

Linwood J. Lewis

Portrayals of Black[1] men during National African American Heritage Month have always been an interesting but conflicted issue for me. As an armchair student of history, and because of my professional interest as a Black developmental psychologist, I know that how Black men are represented is important. Each February, loving and positive portrayals of figures such as Martin Luther King, Jr, Booker T. Washington, W.E.B. DuBois, Paul Robeson, and Frederick Douglass are revered by all Americans as African American history is explored in many of the nation's schools. These positive portrayals in the nation's classrooms are a welcome advance, particularly when one realizes that it has only been fifty years since Black students were legally allowed to enter these classrooms. Unfortunately, these positive February portrayals are juxtaposed against omnipresent media depictions of Black men as criminals, mack daddies, and urban sexual predators. Adolescent males that I have worked with do not describe the sexual aggressiveness that popular culture often portrays, but they are impacted by these images and ideas. My research with Black and Latino adolescent males examines their emotional and psychological experiences related to sexual activity. My work also focuses on how Black and Latino male adolescents' beliefs and expectations about their sexual lives are influenced by their social environments.

Keeping it in perspective

Stereotypes of Black male sexuality in general, and Black adolescent male sexuality in particular, abound in popular culture. Reality TV shows as well as print and broadcast news present ethnic minority crime at much higher rates than nonminority crime—so much so that the cliché of the "perp walk" has become the first introduction to ethnic minority youth for many viewers across the United States. Hypermasculinized, misogynous images and lyrics are produced for mass consumption on MTV by hip hop music producers and have become more prevalent over the past fifteen years.

Matthew Henry, in "He *is* a 'bad mother *$%§!#': *Shaft* and contemporary black masculinity," writes that the 1971 film *Shaft* and its remake in 2000 demonstrate how hypermasculine portrayals of Black men have increased over time. According to Henry, the first *Shaft*—from Isaac Hayes's singing how Shaft is "the Black private dick who's a sex machine to all the chicks" to the double entendre of his name—is a movie obsessed with the phallus. Yet the first *Shaft* weaves in elements of social movements, particularly the Black Power movement, as well as scenes of romance largely missing in the remake. It is clear that the original John Shaft is a lover as well as a fighter. In contrast, contemporary images of Black hypermasculinity emphasize an urban aesthetic of physical prowess and strength. Respect comes through the imminent threat or use of violence and misogyny, avoiding sentimental ties to lovers and promoting a particular kind of sexual aggressiveness. This sexual aggressiveness focuses on the ability to "get some" while steering clear of emotional entanglement and remaining true to one's "boyz."

Of course, media representations of Blacks are more complex than simply hapless criminals running from the police on *Cops* or the latest gangsta video on MTV. But as youth move through puberty toward adulthood, the media and the cultural beliefs they reflect clearly have an important influence on adolescent behavior. How do Black male adolescents negotiate sexual development in a place where Black men are stereotyped as instinctually skilled lovers as well as powerful, violent, misogynic, and sexually aggressive hustlers?

In my work as a research psychologist, I've interviewed a number of urban Black and Latino male adolescents between fourteen and eighteen years old. In order to assess how these youth understood their sexuality, I began by asking nineteen of them to describe their thoughts and feelings about sex, as well as their sexual development over time. After analyzing a series of extensive interviews with these adolescents, I found that these young men are very willing to talk about sex and sexual matters. Although they may not have a formal, academic vocabulary to describe the racial, gender, and sexual complexities they encounter, their stories do turn the cultural stereotypes of Black male sexuality upside down.

Sexual aggression?

Most of the youth in my study said that they, along with their friends, had whistled and yelled sexually suggestive statements at adolescent girls. Many of them explained, however, that their first encounter with sexual intercourse happened when the girl took control. Joseph* described:

> I was in her house, whatever, turning on her computer when she starts undressing . . . And then she kissed me. So I kissed her back. And she was like trying to take it further. (Eighteen years old, Black/Spanish.)

Ricky*, a fourteen-year-old African American boy, relayed something similar:

> She pulls down my pants and then I was like what are you doing and I don't know what the heck she was saying. She was drunk and stuff. Then she put a condom on me and then she just started.

These experiences clearly don't match the hypermasculine stereotypes of sexually assertive Black males that have become so prevalent in US culture. Furthermore, the youth I worked with did not consider the girls' making the first move to be wrong. Instead, they considered sexual activity to be a normal activity for both males and females. It was okay for either to initiate sexual activity in private. When adolescent girls violated age norms in pursuing older sexual partners, however, they were rejected by these youths as "hos" and "chickenheads." Here, the double standard was at work: the older partners of these girls were not stigmatized by having sex with younger girls.

---

*Names changed to protect privacy.

What are youth saying?

When I asked why they had sex, all the youth in my research group said it felt good physically. But many of them also described emotions and the importance of having a close relationship. Henry* came to the interview thugged out, in a football jersey and baggy jeans. He told me about his love for his girlfriend who is, he said, "always there for me." Finding someone who is "there for me" was an important and recurring theme among these young men. They also reported strong positive relationships with girls and women in their lives, both family and friends. Finally, youths described how they had changed as they got older and how their behaviors and beliefs had changed with them. Older youths, between sixteen and eighteen years old, compared their current attitudes toward their partner (respectful and monogamous) to their more promiscuous and uncaring behavior when they were young. Older youths were less influenced by peer pressure, and they remarked on how this same peer pressure had had a lot more impact when they were younger. I found that the younger, less experienced guys bought more of the cultural stereotypes of Black hypermasculinity than their older peers. All in all, the experiences, beliefs, and emotions these youth described show that they must juggle contradictory expectations from parents, peers, and their own ideas about sexuality and masculinity.

During the course of this research, it also became clear to me that politicians, researchers, and the media often misunderstand and misrepresent the beliefs of ethnic minority youth. For example, Jackie*, a nineteen-year-old college student commenting on my research, explained that listening to gangsta rap and watching rap videos does not mean that you believe in the misogyny and violence they represent. She felt that these were entertainment, similar to video games, and not to be taken seriously. Many cultural studies of Black humor agree with Jackie. Mel Watkins, author of *On the Real Side: A History of African American Comedy*, describes "snapping" or the "dozens" (rapid-fire insults directed at friends or others in public) as entertaining, rather than insulting as many earlier commentators on Black life have mistakenly related. In "Looking for the 'Real' Nigga: Social Scientists Construct the Ghetto," Robin D.G. Kelley describes how urban African American life has been homogenized by social scientists. Social scientists in search of "authentic" Black culture were doomed to follow their pre-conceptions and oversimplify the complexity of people's lives. Unfortunately, cultural misapprehensions and stereotypes originating in high prestige sources, like the media and academic research, have real teeth and can cause lasting harm.

What is the media saying?

One example of this damage is the rape case of a Central Park jogger. In 1989 five African American and Latino adolescents were arrested for the brutal beating and rape of a white female investment banker who was jogging in New York's Central Park. Police picked up the adolescents in the park, although no physical evidence linked them to the crime. Media frenzy ensued, with tabloid newspapers referring to the five as a "wolfpack." Donald Trump paid $85,000 for full page ads in *The New York Times* demanding the death penalty if the adolescents were convicted. The unstated and underlying assumption was that these "dangerous urban sexual predators" were clearly capable of such a crime—a belief that was bolstered by many years of stereotyping. Once the young men confessed, their confession was taken at face value despite evidence of coercion.

Contrast this case with the rape of a white female high school student in suburban Glen Ridge, New Jersey. In 1989 four white high school athletes raped their mentally handicapped classmate in a basement. But instead of calls for the death penalty, these young men received considerable support from their community and from the tabloid press in New York City. According to Bernard Lefkowitz's book *Our Guys: The Glen Ridge Rape and the Secret Life of the Perfect Suburb*, the assumption was that nice, middle-class, suburban, white athletes could not possibly have raped their mentally handicapped classmate with, among other objects, a broomstick. In other words, unlike the "wolfpack" in Central Park, they were presumably incapable of such atrocities. The athletes received bail, and although they were ultimately convicted of sexual assault, they got suspended sentences and probation. After all, to convict them of such a crime would ruin their lives.

The press, perhaps inadvertently, has a hand in these cases. Bakari Kitwana, in *The Hip Hop Generation: Young Blacks and the Crisis in African American Culture*, argues that tabloid reporters, without knowledge of adolescent youth culture, misused terms. In the Central Park case, the media made much of the term "wilding"—supposedly, a widely used term for gang rape among New York City's ethnic minority youth cultures. No evidence suggests that this term ever existed. By repeating the term "wilding," the media implied that there was an organized culture of Black-Latino gang rape. No doubt, this misconception contributed to the conviction of these youths. In 2003 the verdicts condemning the Central Park youth were overturned. DNA evidence and a confession from a serial rapist who had raped a woman in a similar manner two days before the Central Park rape absolved the youth, but not until they had served many years in prison. Despite similarities between the Central Park case and a previous rape, police ignored this connection and prosecuted the five adolescents. The serial rapist went on to rape four more women, killing one, after the Central Park incident. He is currently serving thirty-three years to life in prison.

Histories of "dangerous" sexualities

The perception that urban Black adolescents are sexually dangerous is not new. Disenfranchised communities, such as the poor and ethnic minorities, have long been demonized with this narrow view in places such as the United States and United Kingdom. In *Dangerous Sexualities*, Frank Mort writes that during the nineteenth century the sexuality of the urban poor was considered a moral danger, supposedly corrupting upstanding citizens. According to this logic, the poor threatened racial purity. African slaves, whose humanity was called into question in order to justify their enslavement, were cast as animals. Their sexual needs were like other animals, unrefined by civilization and requiring governmental control—supposedly for their own good as well as for the good of society.

John D'Emilio and Estelle Freeman, in *Intimate Matters: A History of Sexuality in America*, illustrate how formal and informal social controls over racial and ethnic minority sexualities have been a part of the United States for 400 years. Miscegenation laws were used to formally prevent sexual interactions between whites and non-whites. Informal controls have included lynching, such as the 1955 murder of Emmett Till, a fourteen-year-old Black adolescent killed in Mississippi for saying "Bye, baby" to a white female store clerk. Such killings were often defended as protecting white women from the sexual predations of Black men, although there was often little or no evidence of sexual behavior on the part of these men.

There are consequences when we construct Black male sexuality in particular ways: these beliefs, stereotypes, and media representations affect the way Blacks are treated. While the adolescent males with whom I have worked do not describe the sexual aggressiveness that popular culture often portrays, clearly, they are impacted by these images and ideas. Psychologists, judges, and other commentators of Black youth culture must get it right. It is past time to understand ethnic minority lives and sexuality in more complex ways and to portray that complexity over the entire year.

Note

1   The use of the term Black, a racial signifier, masks the grouping of diverse ethnic groups of African descent under one banner. I use the term African American here to identify persons who self-identify with African ancestors who were involuntary immigrants to the United States. This is in contrast to voluntary immigrants such as Afro-Caribbeans, who were involuntary immigrants to their own country but who have immigrated to the United States voluntarily. This distinction is especially important because some Afro-Caribbeans hold themselves in contradistinction to African Americans, who are perceived as morally suspect, lazy, and sexually undisciplined. Cultural differences abound across groups that may be perceived as racially monolithic but are ethnically and, thus, culturally diverse.

References

D'Emilio, J., and E. Freeman. 1988. *Intimate Matters: A History of Sexuality in America*. New York: Harper & Row.

Henry, M.A. 2004. "He *is* a 'bad mother *$%@!#'*: *Shaft* and contemporary black masculinity." *African American Review* 38(1): 1–9.

Kasinitz, P., J. Battle, and I.M. Miyares. 2001. "Fade to black? The children of West Indian immigrants in South Florida." *Ethnicities: Children of Immigrants in America*, eds. A. Portes and R. Rumbaut. 267–300. Berkeley, CA: University of California Press.

Kelley, R.D.G. 2004. "Looking for the 'real' nigga: social scientists construct the ghetto." *That's the Joint! The Hip-Hop Studies Reader*. New York: Routledge.

Kitwana, B. 2002. *The Hip Hop Generation: Young Blacks and the Crisis in African American Culture*. New York: Basic*Civitas* Books.

Lefkowitz,. B. 1997. *Our Guys*. New York: Vintage.

Mort, F. 2000. *Dangerous Sexualities: Medico-moral Politics in England Since 1830*. London: Routledge.

Watkins, M. 1994. *On the Real Side: A History of African American Comedy*. New York: Simon & Schuster.

4   Homophobia and harassment in school-age populations

Christine E. Pettett

It was midafternoon and I had just completed interviewing an expert on homophobia in America's schools. I walked outside and saw that the neighborhood convenience store was filling up with its daily crowd of high school students. A boy of about fifteen shouted across to one of his peers—"Hey faggot!"

This kind of teasing, which centers on insulting someone's sexuality or gender presentation, happens daily in schools across the country. According to a year-long Des Moines, Iowa study (www.youth.org/loco/PERSONProject/Alerts/States/Iowa/slurs.html), high school students hear anti-LGBTQ (lesbian, gay, bisexual, transgendered, and questioning) slurs an average of once every seven minutes in a typical school day. More than half of teens surveyed in 2002 by the National Mental Health Association (NMHA) said classmates use terms such as "fag" and "dyke" on a daily basis—and not just to refer to LGBT students. Three of four students targeted for harassment are straight.

According to Laura Lockwood, director of the Trinity College Women's Center and founder of the Trinity Safe Zone program for LGBTQ students, name-calling is the most common form of anti-gay sentiment in schools. Lockwood expresses particular concern about, not just the presence of homophobic insults, but also the "ease with which students use terms like 'gay,' 'dyke,' and 'fag' casually" to register displeasure or banter with classmates without an awareness that doing so might be hurtful or offensive.

Verbal harassment is not an innocuous form of mischief. In the book *We Don't Exactly Get the Welcome Wagon: The Experiences of Gay and Lesbian Adolescents in Child Welfare Systems*, Gerald P. Mallon documents that "verbal harassment causes as much hurt as physical violence because it profoundly damages self-esteem." Slurs and verbal sexual harassment seriously impair mental health and increase rates of depression, suicidal thoughts (and actions), anxiety disorders, and isolation among its victims. Harassment is also linked to poor school attendance, tardiness, inflated dropout rates, and declines in academic performance. Anti-LGBTQ slurs bear a causal relationship to impaired academic opportunity for all students, none of whom are immune to the teasing and stress that homophobic school environments foster.

The nonprofit organization Human Rights Watch (HRW) estimates that two million US students are bullied every year because they are, or are thought to be, homosexuals. A 2001 HRW study of 140 LGBTQ students found that all of those interviewed witnessed or experienced incidents of verbal harassment and other forms of nonphysical harassment, such as written notes, whispered rumor campaigns, obscene telephone calls, graffiti scrawled on walls or lockers, or suggestive cartoons and pornography. Students are no strangers to physical assaults and violence as well. For example, young lesbians and bisexual girls are more than twice as likely as heterosexual girls to be touched or grabbed in a sexual way, and four times as likely to have experienced physical sexual harassment including rape, according to the HRW report "Hatred in the Hallways: Violence and Discrimination Against Lesbian, Gay, Bisexual and Transgendered Students in US Schools" (www.hrw.org/reports/2001/uslgbt/toc.htm).

Forced sexual contact is not the only form of physical assault experienced by those who are, or are perceived to be, LGBTQ. Students also report having their clothing torn, and being spit upon, shoved, slammed into lockers, cut, hit by broken bottles and other thrown objects, and pushed or dragged down stairwells. The NMHA reports that one third of gay students are physically harassed due to their sexual orientation and one in six is beaten badly enough to need medical attention. A number of national social welfare and advocacy organizations—including the National Education Association (NEA), Centers for Disease Control (CDC), HRW and the NMHA, as well as groups specifically oriented towards LGBTQ issues, such as GLSEN (Gay, Lesbian and Straight Education Network), PFLAG (Parents, Families and Friends of Lesbians and Gays), and NYAC (National Youth Advocacy Coalition)—advocate developing tolerance and diversity curricula. However, school board members, administrators, counselors, and teachers do not always greet such initiatives favorably. Leif Mitchell, Northeast member of the GLSEN National Board of Directors and author of the report *Tackling Gay Issues in School*, notes with regret that "too often, teachers do not intervene when they see homophobia in action." Similarly, the 1997 Des Moines study found that fully 93 percent of the time, teachers ignored incidences of LGBTQ insults and harassment.

By and large, the failure of many teachers and counselors to serve lesbian, gay, bisexual, and transgender youth originates from a lack of training. Advocacy groups and educators who support the inclusion of gender expression and LGBTQ identities in tolerance programs assert that prejudice and harassment can only be dispelled by talking directly and frankly about the issue and providing resources for in-school mentoring and support. For example, Lockwood's Safe Zone program incorporates a training module in which members of the college community learn to be sensitive to LGBTQ bias on campus and to provide resources to bias victims. GLSEN has developed another strategy, a teacher training program and advocacy campaign to "make anti-LGBTQ harassment unacceptable within the next three years," reports Mitchell.

One of the most effective strategies to reduce LGBTQ bias in schools is through the development of Gay–Straight Alliances, or GSAs. GSAs are student groups that build support networks among students to address the systematic verbal and physical bullying that students encounter on a daily basis. As an extracurricular activity in public schools, GSAs are entitled to receive equal access to school resources just like all other kinds of nonacademic clubs.

Despite evidence that students are increasingly able to confront and reduce anti-gay bias, not everyone is in favor of such initiatives. Across the country a number of school districts that oppose such organizations have opted to abolish all extracurricular activities rather than permit GSA activity. Actions such as these not only deprive students of the opportunity to build anti-harassment coalitions but may, in fact, create a backlash and exacerbate ill will toward LGBTQ students and their allies.

Some socially conservative groups argue that programs designed to protect LGBTQ youth repress those who believe nonheterosexual behavior is morally wrong. This sentiment is particularly evident in recent debates over Safe Schools initiatives, designed to prevent school violence of the kind that happened at Columbine High School in Colorado (in which the student shooters were known to have been repeated victims of bullying that included frequent use of homophobic insults).

According to a *Wall Street Journal* report, "conservative groups say the safe-schools effort has become a vehicle to promote homosexuality." Karen Holgate, a conservative activist, believes that "gay-rights advocates 'have very cleverly come in under the guise of something that sounds wonderful, and they are promoting another agenda.' School officials and program advocates say they haven't seen similar objections to discussions of bullying based on race, religion or ethnicity." Nonetheless, following objections to LGBTQ-support initiatives in public schools, funding has been withdrawn from many programs designed to combat student harassment.

Furthermore, current federal budget proposals to divert funding from public to private schools through the use of vouchers, such as the Bush administration's "No Child Left Behind," have been of particular concern to LGBT advocates, such as GLSEN Director of Public Policy Mary Kate Cullen. "Faced with the choice of a private school that doesn't ensure a discrimination-free learning environment or a system of public education that is further depleted of much needed funding, LGBT students and their families stand to lose".

In the United States 75 percent of people committing hate crimes are under age thirty, and one in three of these are under eighteen. Educating LGBT youth and straight students about homophobia and its detrimental effects has the potential to transform school culture and create positive change for all minorities in the future. When bias of any kind is condoned in the learning environment, it teaches young people that division and prejudice is appropriate behavior to model. On the other hand, policies and practices that demonstrate tolerance teach young people to uphold the civil rights and basic humanity of all individuals. Today, our schools acknowledge that it is not only inappropriate to condone harassment of ethnic minorities and disabled students, but that doing so has a detrimental effect on the learning environment and the development of a more tolerant society. Organizations like HRW, GLSEN, NEA, and others are currently engaged in a struggle to achieve the same parity for LGBTQ students and those who support them.

References

Mallon, G.P. 1998. *We Don't Exactly Get the Welcome Wagon: The Experiences of Gay and Lesbian Adolescents in Child Welfare Systems*. New York: Columbia University Press.
Mitchell, L. (ed.). 1999. *Tackling Gay Issues in School: A Resource Model*. Stamford, CT: The Gay, Lesbian, and Straight Education Network of CT and Planned Parenthood of Connecticut.

5 Citizenship lessons

Sexuality education in the United States

Jessica Fields and Celeste Hirschman

Contemporary debates over school-based sexuality education are about more than just whether young people should learn about contraceptives, disease prevention, or abstinence-until-marriage. School-based sexuality education is a highly contested arena in the contemporary struggle over heterosexuality and citizenship in the United States.

As school boards, teachers, young people, parents, and legislators argue over whether, what, and when young people should learn about sexuality in school, they are also struggling over what it means to be a sexual person. They are helping to decide what kinds of sexual behaviors, identities, and decisions are acceptable in their schools, neighborhoods, and towns. They are helping to define "good" sexual citizens by delineating which sexual desires, behaviors, and identities confer the rights and responsibilities of belonging, and which preclude full, legitimate citizenship.

Exclusive federal funding for abstinence-only education makes clear the prevailing government definition of the good sexual citizen. Current funding streams require educators receiving federal support to teach that sexual expression is safe only within the confines of monogamous heterosexual marriage. In this abstinence-only education, conservatives have tied the rights and responsibilities of citizenship to a person's participation in private married heterosexuality. According to these conservative regimes, the public pursuit of any other sexual life is contrary to the interests of the US government. These conservative efforts challenge the citizenship claims of the many straight, lesbian, gay, bisexual, poor, divorced, single-parenting, widowed, cohabiting, and marriage-resisting people living sexual lives in the United States.

Promoting heterosexual marriage

Currently, the federal government spends over $100 million annually on abstinence-only education. Under the 1981 Adolescence Family Life Act (AFLA), the government funds programs that promote chastity as a means to prevent teen pregnancies. An amendment to the 1996 Personal Responsibility and Work Opportunity Reconciliation Act (what many know as "welfare reform") strengthened AFLA's message when it established Section 510(b) of Title V of the Social Security Act. Title V funds abstinence-only programs that promote monogamous heterosexual marriage; all funded programs must adhere to an eight-point definition of abstinence education that sexuality education teachers, administrators, and researchers commonly refer to as "A-H." According to A-H, abstinence educators must teach the benefits of confining sexual expression to heterosexual marriage and emphasize that sexual activity under any other circumstances violates standards of behavior and risks broad physical, psychological, and social harm. Another funding stream, Community-Based Abstinence Education (CBAE) enforces A-H more stringently: while Title V programs must not be inconsistent with any aspect of A-H, CBAE programs must explicitly address each of the definition's eight points.

George W. Bush's administration aims not only to continue funding for abstinence-only education but also to link the receipt of welfare benefits to heterosexual marriage. In the welfare program he proposed early in his administration, Working Toward Independence (WTI), Bush left Title V and the A-H funding guidelines intact and increased the annual federal budget for abstinence-only education to $120.75 million. WTI also included provisions that would require states to provide "family formation and healthy marriage efforts" for welfare recipients.

Heterosexuality and marriage in crisis

Sexuality education has long been tied to sexual morality, and contemporary abstinence-only education is no different. The Bush administration promotes abstinence-only education even while admitting that, to date, there has been no research able to demonstrate that abstinence-only education reduces teen pregnancies, delays first intercourse, or prevents sexually transmitted infections (STIs). The efforts of the president and his allies don't seem to address these health concerns. Instead, funding for abstinence-only education is part of a broad and concerted effort to reassert heterosexuality's dominance and to reestablish sanctions against those who are sexually active outside marriage.

Ironically, efforts to establish heterosexuality as the official sexuality of the United States reflect the extent to which heterosexuality is changing and may even be in crisis. Traces of the crisis abound. Vermont recognizes civil unions between gay and lesbian couples, Massachusetts has legalized same-sex marriage, and California offers domestic partnerships. *The New York Times* now includes among its wedding announcements descriptions, complete with photographs, of lesbian and gay unions. Television audiences celebrate—and advertisers align themselves with—the gay and lesbian content of shows like *Will and Grace*, *Queer Eye for the Straight Guy*, *Ellen*, *Queer as Folk*, *Six Feet Under*, and *Oz*. In San Francisco a group from the Women of Color Resource Center, wearing wedding dresses and calling themselves "welfare brides," gathered on Valentine's Day 2003 outside the city's busiest transportation hub to protest federal legislation tying welfare benefits to participation in marriage education and counseling programs. The US Supreme Court asserted in its June 2003 *Lawrence* v. *Texas* decision that the civic right to privacy protects homosexual activity. For conservatives, abstinence-only sexuality education is a response to these changes—one way to reassert that sexuality is a private concern and to publicly reestablish the dominance of private married heterosexuality.

Companion efforts include the 1993 institution of the federal "Don't Ask, Don't Tell" policy, in which the US government rejected the possibility that one could acknowledge same-sex desire, in word or deed, and still serve one's country honorably. The government has also refused to acknowledge the partnered lives of gay men and lesbian women: the 1996 Defense of Marriage Act explicitly granted states the right to deny legal recognition to same-sex partnerships. The assault continues with renewed vigor under George W. Bush and a conservative US Congress. In 2002 the US House of Representatives introduced an amendment to the Constitution establishing that

"Marriage in the United States shall consist only of the union of a man and woman." Together with abstinence-only education policies and funding, these governmental acts help to shore up heterosexuality and marriage—institutions in crisis.

Liberatory models of education and citizenship

As researchers concerned with the social and political implications of sexuality education, we advocate shifting the terms of the debate over sexuality education to address directly the agenda of those promoting abstinence-only instruction. Much academic research continues to evaluate sexuality education's effects conventionally by measuring whether or not sexuality education programs lower pregnancy rates, STI rates, and incidences of sexual activity. Researchers, educators, and policymakers need to broaden notions of "effects." We need also to ask: In what ways might the assertion, that sexual activity outside of private marriage is harmful to person and nation, constitute an assault on young people's rights? What are the broad social consequences of instructing young people that those who do not confine their sexual lives to marriage not only defy established sexual standards but also compromise the well-being of their loved ones and their country?

Conservatives have claimed school-based sexuality education as one field in which to promote a national heterosexuality and establish sexual abstinence as a standard for unmarried people. In contrast, progressive educators, policymakers, and activists have largely neglected the citizenship implications of sexuality education. This neglect effectively concedes to conservatives an important site in the struggle over what it means to be a citizen of the United States. We advocate recognizing the citizenship claims at stake in abstinence-only education. We insist upon a model of sexual citizenship that extends the rights and legitimacy of membership to those whose sexual lives do not conform to established standards *and* promotes healthy sexual expression; encourages people to articulate dissent, curiosity, and knowledge; and equips citizens to critique social institutions and practices that enforce sexual conformity.

6 Transmen

Behind assimilation, problems exist

Jamison Green

In popular culture images of awkward, hairy men in dresses are always good for a laugh. Graceful drag queens appear in magazines, films, and television, and serve as mistresses of ceremonies at community events. The media tells us that men may admire them, but if they are tricked into having sex with one, they should be ashamed and disgusted or they may themselves become targets for ridicule.

But mainstream media finds nothing funny, nor particularly glamorous, about female-to-male (FTM) people. Not that there aren't some talented performers, musicians, writers, actors, and even stand-up comics among the FTM transgender population—there are! The public, though, doesn't treat them with the same fascination it has for MTF transgendered people. Perhaps that's because outwardly, FTM people assimilate more easily. In many cases, it's difficult to even imagine that they were ever women.

This invisibility is a powerful factor in the lives of FTM transgendered and transsexual people.

When a female-bodied individual transitions to life as a male, he is usually on a long trajectory. While some people can simply put on men's clothing and pass for male and live full-time as men, and while there are drag kings who enjoy performing as men periodically but who live as women most of the time, once people take on the label of FTM, they are making a physical transition that often takes several years at best. If the transition is well-managed and legally acknowledged, it requires collaboration with the medical profession—and thousands of dollars.

Trying to imagine the motivation that might drive a person to change sex, some theorists have postulated that sexual expression is a primary drive—in this case, the notion being that FTM people want to be men so they can "correctly" have sex with women, or so that they can indulge in sex as a man would do.

This theory is, doubtless, a gross oversimplification. First, the sexuality of FTM people is as varied as that of any other population segment. There are FTM individuals who are heterosexual, homosexual, bisexual, and asexual, though no research exists that adequately estimates any percentages of people occupying each category. FTM people often have very masculine psyches and physiques, but their genital organs are often very different from those of non-transsexual men. Some may have managed to have phalloplasty, or the surgical creation of a penis, but the majority of FTM people have not had the procedure, either because they cannot afford it or because they are not convinced that the practical result is worth the sacrifice.

Whether the object of their sexual attraction is men, women, transsexual women, or other transsexual men, FTM people often struggle with issues of physical inadequacy, or at least the fear that any potential partner would not be interested in their body. Those transmen who have undergone surgical genital reconstruction are often pleased with the results for themselves, but they still may be afraid that others would not find their penises erotic.

This physical difference, with or without surgical reconstruction, is often sufficient to render many FTM people reticent at best, and avoidant at worst, when it comes to initiating sexual encounters. Though sexual drive is probably not a primary motivator for initiating transition, once a man's body and mind are integrated through transition and he feels connected to the body he occupies, he may enjoy sex more than he did before. This seems to be derived from the gestalt of personality integration. In other words, people are better able to enjoy sex when they feel connected to, at home in, and happy with their own body.

Other issues specific to FTM transpeople are socialization as men and access to healthcare. If they intend to function as men as opposed to "in-between," they need to learn expected male behaviors and how to moderate their own behavior so they can manage social situations within an acceptable range of actions. This does not mean learning how to pretend to be male, or learning to reinforce stereotypes. It is the same socialization procedure that young men experience.

There is nothing false or deceptive about learning appropriate social behavior; it is just that society doesn't provide a "place" for adult people to do this while they are also managing adult responsibilities. He must learn the ropes of being male in his cultural environment, whether that environment is determined by his race, his economic situation, his class, and/or his sexual orientation (which may be different from what he anticipated, too!). In addition, the transman must also do what is required to preserve the health of the body he has, even if that body has female internal organs. This may be a daunting prospect if he lives in an area where there is little medical support available for transsexual people.

The documentary film *Southern Comfort* shows the danger of poor healthcare access. It witnesses the last year in the life of a transman who is dying of ovarian cancer because of the fear, bigotry, and ignorance of the medical community where the man lived. Countless transmen are living in the United States right now who are avoiding healthcare because they fear being ridiculed, mistreated, or having their confidentiality violated by insensitive or inexperienced providers or administrators, and insurance plans that specifically exclude services for transsexual people.

There is one other classic story that reflects a potential challenge for transmen, rendered in the feature film *Boys Don't Cry* and the original documentary *The Brandon Teena Story*. This story of rape and murder generated by the discovery of a young transman's still-female body (the actual event took place in Nebraska in 1993) has been experienced countless times by MTF transwomen, such as Gwen Araujo, who was murdered in Newark, California in 2002 after a group of men discovered she was anatomically male.

Violence and murder are the ultimate insults that all transsexual, transgender, and otherwise gender-variant people are forced to anticipate simply because they exist. The efforts to eliminate this threat to trans lives, to improve access to healthcare, and to reduce stigma and increase understanding for all people who are differently gendered or embodied are the reasons behind the educational effort that has inspired the present-day "Transgender Movement."

The present-day movement began in the early 1990s but has roots in the Stonewall Riots of 1969 in New York, when gender-variant people, some presumed to be drag queens and masculine ("butch") lesbians, fought with police alongside gay and lesbian people. Gender-variant people who cross-dressed or changed their sex were excluded from acknowledged participation almost immediately, as gays and lesbians sought to define the terms of their own liberation. They felt they would find more mainstream acceptance if they didn't have too many different types of people in their contingent.

Transsexual people and people who break gender boundaries in various ways began to publish and agitate for civil rights in the early 1990s, led by people as diverse as Leslie Feinberg, Virginia Prince, Riki Anne Wilchins, Anne Ogborne, Sandy Stone, Kate Bornstein, Louis G. Sullivan, Phyllis Frye, and myself, among many others.

As our work continues, we are making society a safer and kinder place not only for gender variant people, but for everyone.

7　The meanings of rape

Ann J. Cahill

Questioning the meaning of rape may appear, at first, to be a ridiculous proposition. Given the advances in our understanding of sexual violence over recent decades, we have, as a society, at least come to the conclusion that rape is a horrific, violent, and damaging crime—one that is not to be tolerated or excused. The problem with this perspective is that it assumes that merely viewing rape as negative is equivalent to counteracting its pervasive sexist effects and ramifications. History shows us that this is not so. Rape has been defined legally in a variety of ways, from theft to a violation of civil rights, and the fact that a society condemns rape does not necessarily indicate that it respects women's sexual or political autonomy.

In US culture, we needed feminism to name rape as a political, systematic phenomenon that has oppressed women in particular. Susan Brownmiller took up the issue in her groundbreaking work *Against Our Will: Men, Women, and Rape*, and a variety of feminist thinkers pursued the topic throughout the 1970s. Catharine MacKinnon reexamined rape in a strikingly different way in *Toward a Feminist Theory of the State*. Since that work, little has been done to deepen our understanding of the phenomenon of sexual violence even though feminist thought has developed increasingly sophisticated analytical approaches. These advances make it possible to render new insights about rape and sexual violence and begin to correct the flaws inherent in previous theories. While recognizing the importance of past theories about rape, we must engage with new tools and new paradigms to arrive at a more complex and nuanced understanding of the role sexual violence plays in the everyday lives of women.

The work of Brownmiller and MacKinnon represent two main branches of feminist thought concerning rape. In many ways, the position of Susan Brownmiller is the one most familiar to contemporary US culture and the one that has had the largest influence on reforms to rape law in the United States. In the pithy formula that has trickled down to our common consciousness, Brownmiller (and other feminists who took up her theory) claimed that rape was about violence, not sex. Brownmiller wanted to demonstrate the sheer folly and utter offensiveness of investigating rape by focusing on, for example, what the victim was wearing or her former decisions regarding her sexual behavior. For Brownmiller rape was a violent instrument of power, situated firmly within a political structure that gave a disproportionate amount of power to men at the expense of women.

Brownmiller's contribution to our understanding of rape and, therefore, our ability to counteract it was certainly crucial. It led to legal prohibitions against considering the victim's clothing as evidence of consent, and it provided opposition to the familiar assumption that raped women "asked for it." Nevertheless, this understanding of rape has significant problems. For one, it tends to define rape as essentially equivalent to other forms of violent assault. Following this logic, many states have done away with rape as a distinct category of crime. Equating rape with other forms of assault seems counterintuitive and contradicts the experiences of many women who have survived rape. The theory also assumes that, although sex was effectively the means of violence, the relevance of sex to the nature of the crime and the experience of the victim is limited and perhaps peripheral. Again, this assumption seems counterintuitive. Finally, Brownmiller's theory explicitly adopts a gender-neutral theory of rape, which, given its emphasis on political inequality, veils the fact that, overwhelmingly, men commit rape against women. Brownmiller's theory, then, while effectively freeing women's sexuality from the culpability found in traditional approaches to rape, nevertheless seems to overlook some crucial aspects of rape.

Catharine MacKinnon's approach to rape can be seen as an inversion of Brownmiller's formula. Rather than seeking to minimize the role of sexuality in the phenomenon of rape and sexual violence, MacKinnon situated rape within the context of compulsory heterosexuality. In MacKinnon's view heterosexuality is a political structure that prohibits female autonomy—and rape is merely one end of the continuum. Thus, the problem with rape is not that it is violence but that it is the natural extension of a sexuality that eroticizes and demands female submissiveness and dependence.

Again, this theoretical move was an important contribution toward furthering feminist understandings of rape. Specifically, it allowed for productive connections to be drawn between different types of sexual coercion, and it helped to explain the difficulty of distinguishing rape from other instances of (hetero)sexual encounters. However, it also presented a host of theoretical and practical difficulties. As many critics of MacKinnon have noted, her theory tends to define women, their desires, their experiences, in fact, their total being, solely in relation to patriarchy. This is a difficult position to defend because it risks making feminism itself a logical impossibility. If women are completely defined by patriarchy, how would any woman or group of women develop the conceptual tools to criticize sexist political structures? Finally, while the notion of a sexual coercion continuum is useful, it also appears to contradict women's experiences, which generally distinguish between rape and pleasurable, desired heterosexual sex.

Both theories fail because they misunderstand the complex relationships among the body, self, and society. While Brownmiller addresses rape as a political problem, she grounds it in biology, claiming that rape happens because it is a biological possibility. This position is highly unpersuasive because there are many biological possibilities that are not political realities. Brownmiller, then, fails to understand the body and sexuality as social and political artifacts. MacKinnon, on the other hand, has an unsophisticated understanding of the capacities of power, seeing them as total and unrelenting. A notion of power that brings with it the possibility of resistance is both more convincing and of greater explanatory strength because women and their experiences of rape (including their various ways of resisting rape, both individually and collectively) cannot be understood as solely defined and limited by patriarchy.

If rape cannot be reduced to "only violence" or "only sex," then we must look to newer feminist concepts. We should use recent feminist work on the concept of embodiment to update our theories of rape—positions that neither reduce women to victims nor deny the relevance of sexuality; positions that recognize the multiple forms that rape can take and the multiple harms it creates; and positions that place the body at the center of the experience of being raped.

By making the body central to subjectivity—and by understanding the body as both a political construct and a biological one—we avoid many of the dichotomies that seem to underlie the theories of both Brownmiller and MacKinnon. Rape should be approached primarily as an embodied experience. This reasoning allows for a critique of models of the self that prioritize nonmaterial aspects of being (the intellect, rationality, etc.) over material aspects, such as the body and its sensations, "physical memory," and the like. Sexuality and politics no longer manifest themselves as discrete arenas of experience as Brownmiller seems to imply. The body is also capable of resistance, and so while individuals may be impacted by patriarchy and heteronormative roles, they are never reducible to them, as MacKinnon seems to hold. We are able, therefore, to claim that sex is a necessary element in rape and sexual violence, and, therefore, we can more readily focus on the particular sexual harms that rape and sexual violence cause to victims.

Emphasizing the bodily nature of rape also helps us to understand the multiplicity of the forms that sexual violence takes. Different persons live through different bodies; this observation leads us to the obvious conclusion that differences among persons (age, race, sexual orientation, class, etc.) will result in strikingly different experiences of rape and its effects. In previous theories these differences were perceived as problematic: If we cannot arrive at a universal understanding of the phenomenon of rape, are we doomed to silence about it? Addressing a diversity of experiences refuses a hierarchy of sexual abuse and avoids universalizing the meaning of rape. Instead, the unique experiences of individuals are allowed to speak for themselves.

Other benefits accrue from approaching rape as an embodied experience. Because rape is experienced differently by men and women, an embodiment approach allows for gender-specific analysis rather than gender-neutral theories, which have erased these distinctions. Since the person is no longer understood as primarily autonomous and independent, but rather as a nexus of interweaving relationships and experiences, we are able to articulate more clearly just how damaging rape can be to a person—and how healing is able to occur. Most importantly, we are able to name a victimization that occurs disproportionately to women without considering them as nothing but victims.

References

Brownmiller, S. 1975. *Against Our Will: Men, Women, and Rape*. New York: Penguin Books.
MacKinnon, C.A. 1989. *Toward a Feminist Theory of the State*. Cambridge, MA: Harvard University Press.

8 A play that looks at rape

A crime against women (and men?)

Leslie Simon

Picture this: four bodies dressed in black on a small partially lit stage, two men and two women, the men in the middle and the women on either side of the men, bodies poised and upright, eyes focused on the audience, a group of people assembled to hear stories of four rape survivors—two women *and* two men.

Is this heresy? How dare a play that deals with a crime primarily perpetrated against women suggest that rape victimizes men and women equally? And, as the play unfolds, we might also ponder, how dare it talk about rape, a crime of power and domination, as if it had anything to do with sex.

Let me tell you how. Let me try to convince you why it works so powerfully.

Drawing the Shades, written by a former rape prevention peer educator April Elliott, is performed by student actors in colleges and universities across the country. It portrays the trauma of sexual assault by telling the stories of four survivors.

I teach women's studies at City College of San Francisco. The first time I saw *Drawing the Shades* performed at a conference about eight years ago, I knew Elliott, who wrote the play in 1993, had created a classic. By interviewing actual rape survivors and listening carefully to their pain and the details of their stories, she succeeded in constructing a moving twenty-minute exploration about the trauma of rape. By allowing Female 1 and 2 and Male 1 and 2 to speak singly and together, with two, three, and sometimes all four voices, the play demonstrates how each story is completely different, yet each experience of trauma chillingly similar.

When we first produced *Drawing the Shades* at City College of San Francisco, one particularly astute student remarked: "Wherever you are on the sexuality and gender map, you can find a situation close, if not exactly equivalent, to your own."

Putting it in context

According to 2002 data from the Bureau of Justice Statistics, approximately 66 percent of sexual assault victims knew their assailant. In other words, the victim knows the perpetrator, perhaps as a friend, lover, neighbor, or even someone she or he has just met at a party or through a mutual friend. The typical rapist is not a stranger on the street jumping out of the shadows on a dark night.

Drawing the Shades stays faithful to these statistics. Three of the four survivors know their assailants. Moreover, the characters, ranging in age from nineteen to twenty-two represent the group most vulnerable to rape: fifteen to twenty-four-year-olds. But whereas half of the survivors in the play are men, in reality women are overwhelmingly the victims of adult rape.

Nationally, approximately 13 percent of rape victims were male in 2002, according to the National Crime Victimization Survey. Meanwhile, San Francisco Rape Treatment and Trauma Recovery Center reports that about 15 percent of the victims it treats are men.

Of course, men may be more reluctant to report rape, and statistics don't account for the male-on-male rapes that occur all too frequently in prisons. Nonetheless, from our best estimates, we know that an adult female has a much greater chance of becoming a rape victim than an adult male does.

Take note, though, Elliott never intended for the play to stand by itself. An eight-minute video following the performance clearly indicates that among the adult population women are targetted far more than men. But instead of frightening her audiences with grim rape statistics, Elliott wants them to feel compassion for rape survivors. And they do.

Female 1's story is the most typical. She is a straight woman raped by a straight man who wants a sexual relationship with her but with whom she only wants to be friends. Male 1, a bisexual man, has a crush on a man who ends up raping him. Female 2 is a lesbian, gang raped along with her female lover after coming out of a bar; she represents rape by a stranger. Finally, Male 2 is raped by a woman. Although he is sexually interested in her, he makes clear to her that he wants to go slower and postpone sexual intercourse until they get to know each other better. This character could have been the play's undoing. Instead, Elliott's bravery in telling his story moves the piece from mere rhetoric to provocative drama.

In the end, *Drawing of Shades* is a play that teaches us much more than one based solely on statistics would. It looks at a situation that, though less common than other types of rape, is a similarly painful experience. According to Paul Isley, who has studied adult male sexual assault, male victims experience the same reactions to rape as female victims, which include depression, anger, guilt, self-blame, and sexual dysfunction.

Drawing the Shades shows that rape is a violent crime that happens in sexually charged situations. It also demonstrates that violence, a major component of rape, is not inherent in heterosexual relationships, as some radical feminists have argued. Female 1, the only heterosexual woman in the play, knows the difference between sex she wants and sex she doesn't want.

Gender roles

In "The Politics of Sexual Violence" class that I teach, we analyze the political, social, and psychological causes of sexual violence. We look at hierarchical systems of power that grant privileges to certain groups of people while denying them to others. Privileged groups—such as whites, men, and heterosexuals—can discriminate and perpetrate violence against nonprivileged groups, as was seen in the United States when white male slave owners systematically raped black women.

We also examine the role of social conditioning in the perpetuation of violence, such as the gender roles in our culture that encourage men to be aggressive and women to be passive. Finally, we study how an insecure person, who has been granted powers and privileges, may resort to violence as a means of boosting an unstable ego. In their book *You Can Be Free: An Easy-To-Read Handbook for Abused Women*, Ginny NiCarthy and Sue Davidson put it this way: "He's afraid he's weak, so he acts tough."

To fight rape, we need to make political and social changes so that power and wealth are not concentrated among an elite group that perpetuates a system of abuse in housing, jobs, healthcare, education, and social relations. But we also need to stop perpetuating the psychological conditions that foster abusive behavior. If children grow up in loving homes where they are not subject to physical, sexual, and/or emotional abuse, they will become healthy, secure adults not prone to inflicting their pain on people weaker than themselves.

We need to care about boys and men as potential victimizers of rape. And as *Drawing the Shades* teaches us, we need to care about women—and men—be they straight, gay, or bisexual, as potential victims of rape.

9 The "down low"

New jargon, sensationalism, or agent of change?

Gilberto R. Gerald

Mounting anxiety about sexual encounters with high-risk partners spotlights hush-hush concern—Laura Randolph, "The Hidden Fear: Black Women, Bisexuals and the AIDS Risk," *Ebony*, 1988.

Long before being on the "down low" became part of the vernacular, Laura Randolph, a writer for *Ebony,* sought to illustrate that black women are unwittingly at risk for HIV through sexual relations with men who lead secret sexual lives with other men. To demonstrate the point, Ms Randolph provided an inaccurate account of how an HIV/AIDS prevention activist had put the lives of black women in jeopardy. I was *that activist.*

It was clear to me and others, once the article was published, that Ms Randolph needed an example of a man on the "downlow" (or "DL") and that any black man who admitted having sex with other men as well as with women would do. In my case, a simple line of inquiry would have revealed that I was an unsuitable representative of what she had hoped to show in her article. In reality, I had engaged in vaginal sex nearly nine years prior to the emergence of the AIDS epidemic. The sexual exchange was with an Asian woman and it involved the use of condoms to prevent conception.

Fast forward to 2003 and 2004 and there is again media hype about an old issue, this time with a new hook—the term "down low." Thankfully, the media no longer needs a substitute for the real subject of concern. J.L. King, author of *On The Down Low: A Journey Into the Lives of "Straight" Black Men Who Sleep with Men*, was not only willing to write about the issue from firsthand experience but also willing to appear on *The Oprah Winfrey Show* in 2004. The episode's title was "A Secret Sex World: Living on the 'Down Low.'" Several major newspapers also featured men on the "DL," including *The New York Times Magazine*, which ran an August 2003 cover story written by Benoit Denizet-Lewis entitled "Double Lives on the Down Low."

Living on the "DL" is but one of several terms in a broader arsenal of code language that is in constant flux. The term serves to describe a specific sexual interest and a shared sensibility among individuals and groups in the black community about male-to-male sexuality and black manhood. These sensibilities are, more often than not, distinct from sensibilities held by black men and by non-black men who identify themselves as gay. Men on the "DL" may have sex with men but they do not relate to the established gay community, and, rather than coming out, they choose to keep their sexual activities private—in other words, on the "down low."

The recent attention in the media to black men on the "DL" makes it appear as though this is a new development in black male behavior. Further, it suggests that this behavior differs essentially from behavior found in other racial or ethnic groups. This current public discourse shows a lack of knowledge of earlier concern with the issue, leaving solutions to the HIV/AIDS epidemic among the African American population unexplored and unsupported. Culturally grounded HIV-prevention models based on evidence of effectiveness in the black community are lacking, and a deeper understanding of the factors that contribute to risk behavior in black men and women is needed.

Beyond the talk

In 1986, long before the term "DL" came into common use, the now defunct National Coalition of Black Lesbians and Gays (NCBLG) carried out one of the earliest efforts to address HIV/AIDS within the black community. NCBLG developed a nationally distributed HIV-prevention brochure that included the term "men who go both ways," code language that had currency in some quarters of the black community at the time, along with other terms such as "In the Life," which is the title of Joseph Beam's 1986 groundbreaking anthology of essays by black gay writers and artists. NCBLG and others engaged in HIV prevention incorporated these terms and other language into their work to recognize the large community of black men who slept with other men but would never identify with the word "gay" or with gay culture.

While it is important to examine changing jargon, the bigger issue, since the beginning of the epidemic, is that research to support effective HIV prevention for blacks is sorely needed. In the midst of this media focus on the "DL," the Centers for Disease Control and Prevention (CDC) embarked in late 2003 on a new initiative to provide multiyear funding for community-based efforts to stop the spread of HIV. The CDC required that applicants for grants use one or more of the interventions included in the Procedural Guidance, which catalogued evidence-based intervention models that the CDC had endorsed as effective. For organizations interested in providing targeted outreach and health education/risk reduction to high-risk, non-gay identified black men, picking a model from the CDC menu was challenging. While the Procedural Guidance described processes for adapting and tailoring models to meet the needs of specific populations, only one of the CDC models, Community Promise, was specifically described as having been tested among non-gay identified men who have sex with men.

The paucity of CDC endorsed models that have been researched and developed for use in the diverse groups of black men at high risk for HIV infection or transmission is not surprising. In light of the need for more effective approaches, researchers are saying more study is needed. This need should enter into the public discourse to promote the development and dissemination of effective models.

In the February 2004 issue of the *Journal of Black Psychology,* Vickie Mays, Susan Cochran, and Anthony Zamudio call for a renewal in public funding for research that examines how social, interpersonal, and community contexts factor into HIV risk taking. This article also identifies best practices in mental health interventions for black men who have sex with men and measures sexual orientation and behavior in studies involving large numbers of the black population.

Similarly, in a paper published in the same issue of the *Journal of Black Psychology,* Lula Beatty, Darrell Wheeler, and Juarlyn Gaiter recommend:

> using and developing, if necessary, well-articulated theories appropriate to the culture and experiences of the African American population to guide research;

acknowledging and controlling for diversity of the African American population [as part of research], especially in regard to factors that are associated with HIV/AIDS . . . ; [and] conducting more studies on structural interventions that investigate how sociopolitical and environmental factors shape and can effectively change health behaviors in African American communities.

It remains to be seen if the attention recently given to black men on the "DL" represents just another spike in sensational media attention to the issue of HIV/AIDS in blacks—or a turning point spawning renewed and expanded community action and scientific research.

10 Teaching and learning

Latina sociology of sex

Gloria González-López

Recent US census figures confirmed a phenomenon that I have been anticipating for some time. The changing demographics show that Latinos make up the largest minority group in the United States (37 million). According to one study, Latinos represent the majority of births in California. As I reflect on these statistics, I return to the ways in which these demographics impact the study of human sexuality in the United States. I am also reminded of why I first began to conduct sexuality research with Latino immigrant populations.

In the fall of 1995, I led a Latina adult women's support group in Los Angeles as part of my clinical training as a therapist. For many women in the support group, this was their first opportunity to explore their emotional lives in a safe atmosphere with other adult women. Over the course of eight weekly meetings, women in the group developed deep bonds with each other and with me as their group facilitator. They expressed a desire to explore the most intimate details of their lives as women. However, they remained surprisingly silent about one issue: their sex lives.

When I questioned the women in the group about this silence, they immediately asked whether they *could* discuss their intimate experiences and their sexual lives. The sessions became intense and their sexual concerns seemed endless. During our group sessions, we explored countless issues involving virginity, orgasm and sexual satisfaction, relationships, homosexuality (gay and lesbian), sexual practices, reproduction and sex, sexual fantasies, extramarital affairs, prostitution, sexually transmitted diseases, sexual morality, machismo, as well as their concerns about providing sex education for their children.

Some women felt secure about sharing experiences of sexual victimization (rape and incest), while others disclosed their deepest sexual fears, such as becoming a lesbian. These dialogues around sexuality enhanced the quality of our discussions and extended the longevity of the group, which continued for an extra eight months. While the life of the group was extended, it seemed relatively short compared to the women's curiosity and desire to learn as much as possible about sexuality. What was so powerful about the sex lives of these women? Why, originally, was there so much silence around these issues?

When I began my doctoral program in sociology, very few of these issues were adequately addressed. In my graduate seminars on sex, gender, and feminist studies, there was a glaring lack of attention to Latina sexualities. On the other hand, the women in the group had endless questions about sexuality, which they put in the context of gender, class, race, citizenship, language, religion, and other social factors. Cultural difference, inequality, socioeconomic segregation, and social injustice had shaped their views of sexuality and reproductive health. These factors also influenced the kind of sex education they were providing for their children. However, these concerns were rarely a part of my academic training.

Witnessing the social process that shaped the sex lives of the women in the group, I embarked upon my own personal transformation. The group compelled me to revisit my well-considered professional plans, and I chose to begin research on the sex lives of Mexican immigrant women. This was only the beginning of a never-ending quest to investigate and draw attention to the sexual lives of Latina women.

It has been some time since I led the Latina group, but I continue to learn about sexuality from the Latina women with whom I interact. Now as a professor teaching an undergraduate class entitled "Chicana/Latina Sexuality," I realize that part of my motivation to teach the class arises from my own unresolved issues. I wanted to teach the class that I would have liked to take eight or nine years ago.

Enthusiastic and prepared with an extensive reading list of Chicana/Mexicana sexuality research, I still encountered a challenge. How would I teach a group of mostly young Chicanas about Latina sociology and sex?

I have always known that passion is an inevitable part of sexuality. Blending pedagogy and passion seemed like a good combination for the course. Following one of the most admired apostles of education in Latin America, Paolo Freire, I opted for a form of education that would aim toward freedom, justice, and change. From day one I invited my students to emotionally engage the reading material. Beyond thinking about Chicana/Latina sexuality, I invited students to start *feeling* about Chicana/Latina sexuality. During class discussions, we navigated differences in the ways in which Chicanas and Mexicanas shaped their sexual lives. In learning about the history of Chicana and Mexicana sexualities, I encouraged students to imagine back through history to the collective experiences of women who were raped—a history that shaped the conquest of California and the southwestern United States. This dynamic is also mirrored by more recent atrocities in Ciudad Juárez, Mexico. The testimony of a Chicana lesbian, who volunteered to speak to the class, illustrated the social and cultural forces involved in freely embracing her sexuality and the difficulties of attempting to come out.

As my students and I embarked on this learning journey, "conscientizacão," or the "awakening of consciousness" promoted by Freire, we broadened our understanding of sexuality. The relationship between the feelings surrounding sexuality, alongside the issues that shape Latina sexualities, triggered intense reactions. But it also generated enthusiasm and curiosity. We approached issues through the "nosotras" perspective— a concept proposed by Chicana feminist Gloria E. Anzaldúa. The nosotras approach (nosotras meaning "we, female"; nos meaning "us"; and otras meaning "the other") allows us to place Chicanas and Mexicanas at the center of our discussions and analyses. The nosotras perspective encourages a feminist sociological perspective, emphasizing structural causes of marginalization.

Invariably, my students would ask, "So, how do we challenge all these inequalities? How do we promote social justice and change? How do we reclaim our sexualized bodies? How do we teach Chicanas and Mexicanas to develop gender consciousness with regard to sexuality?"

My experiences have exposed me to the same challenges. Each semester I have different students, but the questions are often the same and equally profound. The questions are also endless, and all of us explore potential answers.

At times I have no choice but to remain silent while listening to the engaging and interesting discussions of students. By the time they identify new themes for future research, a ringing sound indicates that it is time to dismiss our class—interrupting their stimulating debates. After erasing the board and getting rid of the chalk on my hands, I choose to stay after class, alone, by myself. After taking a deep breath, I inevitably go back in time to those years in Los Angeles. Then, the image of those eight women who changed my professional fate appear inside my empty classroom to remind me that their daughters grew up and now attend college. Their daughters are my students. The echo I did not find those years while trying to learn about Latinas and sex I am now finding while doing my very best to both teach and learn from a new generation of Chicana women eager to explore the sociology of Latinas and the intricacies of sex.

11 Christian right rhetoric

Exploring anti-gay politics online

A profile of Janice M. Irvine

Janice Irvine has examined the inner workings of a culture war and seen firsthand the power of propaganda. She has dodged fist fights and endured screaming matches. Her work, at times, has left her depressed.

Irvine studies the Christian right.

Since the 1960s, she says, the right wing has used rhetoric to mobilize communities and gain political clout. One of the group's earliest targets was sex education; their tactic was to spread untruths and demonize sex educators. Depravity narratives—that teachers were taking off their clothes for anatomy classes, that young children were being taught about sodomy—riled otherwise calm individuals.

"We have a culture of sexual shame in general," Irvine says. "The rhetoric of the Christian right taps into that. They don't have to say much to make people scared."

More recently, Irvine, a sociology professor at University of Massachusetts at Amherst, has looked at how conservative Christians direct similar strategies toward sexual rights. Her article, "Anti-Gay Politics Online: A Study of Sexuality and Stigma on National Websites," appears in *Sexuality Research & Social Policy* (Vol. 2, No. 1). For the study, Irvine examined the websites of six groups that were prominent in opposing gay rights—Concerned Women for America, Focus on the Family, the Family Research Council, Traditional Values Coalition, the American Family Association, and Americans for Truth—monitoring and analyzing the content for six months. She found that rather than using extreme stigmatizing rhetoric, as has been done in the past, these groups tended to present biased information as objective news and opinions as scientific argument.

The websites of Traditional Values Coalition (TVC) and Concerned Women for America contained the strongest language, depicting sexuality as degrading or embarrassing, and linking gay men to child molestation and other depraved acts. For example, in September 2003, Irvine points out, TVC featured a story titled "California Congresswoman Proudly Supports Obscene Bisexual Conference"; a summary of the article read, "San Diego Congresswoman Susan Davis (D) attended a bisexual conference over the weekend that featured full female and male nudity and workshops on sex toys." In the same month, the group published two articles online, "North Carolina Homosexual Teacher Arrested on Molestation Charges" and "Two Homosexuals Arrested on Child Molestation Charges," in addition to posting its regular link "Homosexual Child Molesters." TVC describes itself as the largest nondenominational church lobby in the United States with a membership of 43,000 churches.

Focus on the Family, the Family Research Council, and the American Family Association had much less anti-LGBT coverage on their sites, Irvine found, and yet, they are leaders in anti-gay politics. To get their word out, these groups used other media outlets, such as radio, email, and newsletters.

"In November 2003, Massachusetts legalized gay marriage; there was a volatile reaction," Irvine says.

> I expected more use of the Internet for organizing. Focus on the Family sent representatives to Massachusetts and launched a legal challenge, but there was no mention of the issue on their Web site. It seems that some of these organizations are at an early phase in the use of the Internet.

Historically, conservative Christians have been at the forefront of utilizing communications technology to spread their messages and sway politics, according to Irvine's research. In the 1920s and 1930s, she writes, they established radio broadcast ministries. Father Charles Coughlin, who spouted anti-Semitic rhetoric and defended fascist policies on his radio show, reportedly received 80,000 letters weekly in the mid-1930s. Conservative Christians were also quick to realize the potential of television, Irvine writes. Jerry Falwell, a popular televangelist in the 1970s and 1980s, heads The Faith and Values Coalition, a political action committee, and has raised $2.5 billion for his causes.

Today, there are roughly one million online religion websites. Cyber-religion could become the dominant form of religion, according to scholar Brenda Brasher, who is cited in Irvine's study. "If online religion . . . has the capacity to transform the future of religion," Irvine writes, "it will also transform the future of politics, because the escalation of conservative religious political activity has been one of the hallmarks of the late twentieth, early twenty-first century political landscape."

During the past twenty-five years, national Christian right organizations have been the most politically mobilized opponents of LGBT rights. Their rhetoric—calling gay materials pornography or gay men pedophiles—associates lesbians and gay men with negative and frightening meanings, Irvine says.

TVC's online "Homosexual Urban Legends" series is an example of that. One article of that series, "Exposed: The Myth That '10% are Homosexual' Updated," challenges Kinsey's analysis that 10 percent of males are "more or less exclusively homosexual" (rating a five or six on the Kinsey scale). TVC's article cites a National Health and Social Life Survey, which found 2.8 percent of the male population and 1.4 percent of the female population identify as gay, lesbian, or bisexual. TVC's article, however, fails to include data from surveys regarding men and women who reported same-sex behavior and attraction but didn't identify themselves as lesbian or gay. Irvine writes that TVC's article "argued that homosexuals used the 'bogus' figure in order to 'recruit children into the homosexual lifestyle and to lobby for . . . special legal protections for homosexuals.'"

Irvine says:

> The Christian right uses data in a distorted or misleading fashion, much of it based on methodologically problematic studies. The uninformed may be less able to evaluate these seemingly scientific reports, and there is potential for journalists to take this material directly from sites.

Since the election of President George W. Bush, Irvine says, the right wing feels it has been given license to continue and expand its rhetoric.

In the case of marriage equality, conservatives often warn of a domino effect. When the Supreme Court struck down a law banning sex between adults of the same sex, for example, Justice Antonin Scalia's dissent argued that if sodomy laws were illegal, laws against incest and bestiality would become illegal too. The *Village Voice* lampooned his opinion in an article "Petaphilia: The Great American Man–Dog Marriage Panic." Irvine says, "People who want our country to value individual and civil rights, and a quality of openness and freedom, need to be involved in educating people about the problematic rhetorical strategy the right is engaged in and neutralizing it, even through parody."

Irvine's research, which she started more than a decade ago, provides a strong response to Christian right rhetoric. She first became interested in the phenomena during debates in the 1980s and 1990s on sex education. Her book, *Talk About Sex: The Battles over Sex Education in the United States*, was published in 2002.

In 1981, the US Office of Population Affairs began administering the Adolescent Family Life Act, providing funding for what is now known as abstinence-only sex education. "This curriculum showed up in communities and generated huge culture wars," Irvine recalls. "I was living in Cambridge and the surrounding communities were completely coming apart over this. I knew this was the issue to take on."

At one town hall meeting she attended, people were screaming and scuffles were breaking out. Parents were pushing and shoving. One of the organizers got up to speak but collapsed. No one knew what had happened, Irvine remembers. Then, they were informed he had had an anxiety attack. "That has stuck with me. It was emblematic of the intense emotions of that time."

Even under the more liberal Clinton administration, issues of sexuality remained taboo. In 1994, for example, then Surgeon General Joycelyn Elders said at a UN-sponsored conference on AIDS that masturbation "is a part of sexuality, and it's a part of something that perhaps should be taught" as a means to prevent AIDS and as part of comprehensive sex education. Less than two weeks later, Clinton asked for her resignation.

"Clinton fired her and no one spoke out to defend her," Irvine says. "People were afraid of being stigmatized by the right wing as a pervert."

Part 2

www., TV, and sexual commodification

Television and the Internet have at least a couple of things in common. They are both visual mediums, driven by the desire to expedite communication and spread information. They also proliferate sexuality, and in particular, the commodification of sexuality. That is, sex that sells. In sexy survivor shows, *Girls Gone Wild* DVDs, and the exponential rise in the amount of pornography now available online, we can see that sexuality is used to both facilitate more conversations and to sell products. Of course, this is not all that new.

Historically, there have always been controversies about television and sexuality. In the "golden years" of television in the 1950s, married couples on TV were required to have two separate beds. By the 1970s, Mr and Mrs Brady were sharing a super-sized king bed while the rest of the Bunch slept tucked away in their gender-appropriate, shared bedrooms. Certainly, no one would argue that explicit sexual content on TV, both verbal and visual, has risen steadily since then. Indeed, some organizations have devoted themselves to monitoring every show on the air and documenting the instances of sexual material: implied, subtle, or otherwise. As more sexuality shows up on our TV screens, how representative of real people's experience are these images?

If there is more sex on TV—and certainly there is no lack of it on the Internet—what does this mean for society? Social scientists have long debated how the media impacts people's behavior. On the one hand, some have argued that exposure to sexual images effectively programs people to have more sexual desires and to mimic the behavior they see on the screen. Others have argued that people have much more agency, autonomy, or "will" when it comes to viewing sexual scenes (or any scenes for that matter); people can distinguish fact from fantasy and act accordingly. Some would say that the multitude of sexual images now available is simply a mirror for desires that have always existed. These debates continue and promise to increase in intensity as more and more people have access to previously "taboo" images.

Sexual democratization?

In this information age, one thing is for certain: equal access to images of sex and sexuality exist more now than ever before. In the past, it was largely the elite and ruling classes who were able to procure erotic images. Pornography as a genre has existed since the rise of mass media (in the form of print, lithography, photographs, film, and video). But only in the last thirty years have moving images been available to large numbers of the general public. Now, as anyone reading this can attest, just about everyone can find a limitless array of extraordinarily explicit sexual content, visual or in print, live or recorded. This marks a new era for sexuality, when we are privy to more sexual information and images than in any other time in history.

Through technology, there are new realms of possibility for sexual experience and experimentation. We can communicate and meet with people whom we wouldn't have encountered otherwise. How do these forums change the way we, literally, "articulate" our sexuality? As we go through the process of "marketing" ourselves online, describing our physical looks, our fantasies, our preferences—how might this alter the way we feel about ourselves as sexual persons? Are we simply honing our sexual sensibilities as we peddle and profile our sexual wants and attributes? With technologies that can erase any supposed imperfections—in size, color, shape, and age for example—how do online images of others and ourselves impact us as sexual beings? In the 1970s, there were people who regularly posted personal ads in newspapers, looking for love or maybe just looking for a one-night stand. Now, an unprecedented number of people are engaged in a similar process, in more rapid succession than was possible with a print medium. Unlimited access of this kind also spells danger for some. Sexual predators are nothing new, but they now have a superefficient forum in technologies that regularly outstrip law enforcement's monitoring abilities. In this section, consider how media and the commodification of sexuality are linked. What do communications technologies and the massive marketing of sexual images mean in terms of how our sexualities are being shaped on a daily basis? Do these images simply quench a thirst for desires already there, or do these images, online conversations, and encounters actually influence what it is we want from our sexual lives?

12 Surfing for healthy sexualities

Sex and the Internet

Deborah Levine

Do you know the word most often searched for on the Internet? Yes, you're right. It's SEX.

More and more people like you and me are turning to the Internet for sexual health information, entertainment, and romantic rendezvous. Seventy percent of Americans spend time online, according to the 2006 Pew Internet and American Life Project. That's approximately 128 million people, evenly split between men and women. Sixty-six percent of online surfers look for health information; 18 percent search for information on sensitive or embarrassing topics . . . Hmmm, could sex be one of them?

The anonymity of the Internet makes it the perfect place to get accurate sexual health information. From scientific facts and advice to tips and techniques, this information can help you maintain a long-term relationship, make new friends, or even find love and romance.

Think about it: When's the last time you asked a sex question to your doctor? Or talked to your friends about what you and your partner did in bed last night? Or made an appointment with your clergyperson for a frank discussion? The truth is we live in one of the most overtly sexualized societies (look at current movies, music, fashion, advertisements), but until recently we have had few places to find out if what we do behind closed doors is considered "normal." Then along came the Internet.

Since the advent of the Internet, the definition of "normal" has greatly expanded. With its wealth of information, the Internet can alleviate any shame or embarrassment that individuals may have about sexual issues. You can explore your sexual options in the relative safety and obscurity of cyberspace, and if you spend some time surfing, you'll be surprised at the variety, depth, and breadth of what's available.

Research shows that people who discuss sexuality openly and are comfortable with their bodies are better lovers and life partners. Taking advantage of what the Internet offers can provide you with the tools for a satisfying, active sexual life well into your senior years.

Riffraff opinion versus high quality information

Everyone has an opinion and these days you can find many of them online. But if you want facts and science, you need to "look for the union label." In other words, if you go to a sexual health Web site or a site professing sex advice, make sure you click and read the credentials of the person or organization behind the site. Best bets are reputable nonprofit organizations such as The Society of Obstetricians and Gynecologists of Canada, Advocates for Youth, Planned Parenthood or the American Social Health

Association. Other good sources include international governmental organizations such as Health Canada, the US National Institute of Health, or Britain's National Health Service. Universities are another good source of current and correct information.

If you are looking at a private site, click on the link usually found at the bottom of the homepage that says "About Us" or "Who We Are" to find out who's who and what's what. Look for credentialed columnists or an advisory board that reviews the material as well as information such as where and what the people behind the scenes studied. Experts need more than initials such as M.A. or Ph.D. behind their names because while a Ph.D. in mathematics is a wonderful thing, it doesn't qualify someone to write a sex advice column.

Beyond textbook sexuality

If you want to learn about more esoteric sexual practices—from bondage to voyeurism—you can find groups with similar interests on the Internet. Taking a peek at the fringes never hurts and might help open your mind to the myriad of possibilities. Even if you don't end up regularly partaking in an alternative practice, you will have learned in a safe and nonjudgmental way about the sexual possibilities that exist in the world. One way to navigate through fetish and kink sites without being bombarded by spam from commercial pornography producers is to start with Gloria Brame's Kinky Links. Gloria is the coauthor of *Different Loving: The World of Sexual Dominance and Submission*.

We all need variation in our sexual styles, and the Internet is a good place to learn new tips and techniques to keep things exciting. You can find sites that teach everything from giving an erotic massage to pleasuring yourself. And you can get sex-toy recommendations from women, men, and experts at places like Good Vibrations, My Pleasure, or Libida.

Leveling the playing field

No matter what your interests are and what information you seek online, education can help broaden your views of sexuality. The Internet levels the playing field and removes the shame or embarrassment that some people may have about sexual issues. The Internet allows us all to be novices and experts at the same time. You can quietly find things you know nothing about. You can explore sexual fantasies without fear of rejection. You can make mistakes without ever having to see the same people again. You can become an expert in the art of sex and lovemaking without leaving the comforts of home.

Armed with an understanding of the range of sexual expression, your newfound knowledge can serve you well. You can, if you wish, take what you've learned online and translate it into your personal life offline. Or, you can simply leave with greater knowledge about the diversity of human sexuality.

Remember, people who are comfortable with sex are sexy. Let the Internet be your new source of sexual health information, exploration, and education.

13 Sexual networks online

Gregory Rebchook and Alberto Curotto

> The Internet has changed my life . . . it has been like a third parent to me almost . . . I had
> my first sexual experience through someone I met on the Internet. I had my first relationship
> through someone I met on the Internet. I have learned so much about life, and how people
> deal with each other through the experiences I have had through the Internet . . . but it has
> also made me lie . . . because I like someone and I want them to like me so I adapt myself
> to what I think they might like.
>
> (Thirty-seven-year-old bisexual male, interviewed online)

Gay/bisexual men's use of the Internet to meet sex partners has captured the attention
of public health officials, HIV-prevention professionals, community activists, and
researchers alike. The medical literature contains case studies of men who contracted
HIV through unprotected anal sex with men they met online, and syphilis has been
spread through sexual networks of gay/bisexual men that were formed on the Internet.
Focusing solely on the epidemiology of HIV and other sexually transmitted infections
among men who go online to seek out male sexual partners, however, barely scratches
the surface of the transformative effect that the Internet has had on the lives of many
gay/bisexual men.

To gain a broader understanding of the Internet's role in the lives of gay/bisexual
men we obtained research grants from the University of California's AIDS Research
Program and the National Institutes of Health, which enabled us to conduct detailed,
real-time online interviews with over a hundred individuals recruited from chatrooms.
This article relates some of the findings from our analysis of these interviews and
information about participants' sexual behaviors collected in a self-administered online
survey.

The online environment is vast and rich in its diversity and complexity, and no less
so for gay/bisexual men. Countless gay-oriented websites provide access to community
resources; coming out support; education about political and activist initiatives that
are relevant to gay/bisexual men; gay men's health information; opportunities for
socializing and communicating with others facing similar issues, regardless of their
geographic location; and all manners of sex-oriented entertainment—including sites
that eroticize unprotected anal intercourse, also known as "barebacking."

Many websites and online service providers offer a variety of features, often organized
by location and/or special interest, which allow people to communicate with each other
in public chatrooms or via private chats. Chatrooms also provide a convenient way to
identify others who are online at any given moment by looking at the list of everyone
currently in a particular room. People who are looking to expand their social or sexual

networks often browse through these lists and read other users' personal profiles to decide whether or not to contact any of them. Online profiles can contain almost any information someone wants to reveal about themselves, including physical appearance and photographs, sexual orientation, location, relationship information, sexual interests, drug use, HIV status, a potential partner's desired attributes, hobbies, etc. Any subsequent communication may lead to immediate or future in-person meetings, the development of online relationships, and/or sexually explicit online exchanges (sometimes called cybersex) via a chat client or a webcam.

The Internet offers men seeking to meet each other many ways to do so other than chatrooms—from freely accessible e-groups and bulletin boards to websites with personals advertising for everything from long-term relationships or friendships to immediate, no-strings-attached, sexual encounters. An ever growing number of subscription websites provides access to databases of personal profiles so members can search for other subscribers with compatible interests and desires.

The variety of online venues has helped men create new social and sexual networks among men and has provided new settings for sexual encounters. Nearly every respondent in our study reported that, thanks to the Internet, their number of sexual partners and encounters had increased. Many participants described the ease of finding sexual partners in both a positive and negative manner. On the positive side, they generally seemed to appreciate the convenience and directness of cruising online, as well as the wide variety of partners available. Some described the anonymity of online communication as one of the Internet's major advantages over traditional sex-seeking venues, allowing them to avoid hostile or intolerant environments and enabling them to carefully choose which of their personas to present to potential sex partners. On the negative side, many men were frustrated by the lack of more lasting and intimate relationships resulting from these online encounters. Additionally, many participants expressed a concern that the Internet could reveal gay men's sexual lives to a larger straight public, reinforcing conservative heterosexual notions that gay men are overly fixated on sex.

Men in our study had mixed impressions about the relationship between Internet use and risky sexual activity. Some men felt that "if someone is going to be risky they are going to do it with or without the Internet. I think more people are satisfied with the fantasy online." Others felt that the Internet contributes to gay/bisexual men's willingness to engage in unprotected anal intercourse. One respondent said that the Internet "has made 'barebacking' such an acceptable practice," and another reported that the Internet "is making [barebacking] readily available to everyone. I never had heard of it until I got online."

"Hook ups?" Yes. But a whole lot more . . .

Nearly all the men we interviewed reported sexual activity with a man they had met online, and their behaviors regarding unprotected anal sex could be classified into discrete patterns: never having anal sex; always avoiding casual online "hook-ups" and using condoms in other sexual relationships; always using condoms for anal sex *without* any discussion of condoms, HIV, or safer sex; or always using condoms for anal sex *in addition to* discussing each partners' HIV status, HIV testing, and sexual histories, and expressing a desire to stay HIV-negative or to avoid infecting others.

Other men did report instances of unprotected anal sex with someone they met online. Some said that occasionally they had unprotected intercourse with men they met online and that they never discussed HIV or condoms with them. Others said that they used condoms with men they met online, but that they did *not* do so with "known" partners; regrettably, from an HIV-prevention point of view, a "known" partner might simply be someone they met in person more than once without ever discussing sexual risk. Some of the men we interviewed who were not HIV-positive said that they would have unprotected anal sex with someone they met online if he told them he was HIV-negative. Such instances of "serostatus disclosure" were often incomplete since there was no communication about testing or potentially risky sex shortly before, or since, testing. Still others said that they had unprotected sex with men they met online without any discussion of HIV status or condoms unless the partner insisted on condom use. Few participants said they never used condoms, but many men left condom use decisions entirely to their partners.

Whereas the Internet's role in facilitating sexual risk behaviors among gay/bisexual men is still unclear, our interviews have shown that the Internet plays an important and multifaceted role in the lives of the gay/bisexual men in our study. For most men Internet use resulted in increased occasions for sexual encounters, which provided opportunities for risk-taking behavior. However, whether or not these men would have engaged in risk behavior were it not for the Internet was beyond the scope of our study.

Exactly how the Internet does, or does not, contribute to gay men's HIV-risk behavior has not been unequivocally answered. What we did find is that, for many of our participants, the Internet has been a unique and invaluable tool in the development of their sexual identity and self-expression. Most men appreciated the opportunity the Internet offered to socialize and access resources safely and anonymously. Occasionally, men were able to develop and sustain supportive interpersonal relationships, and sometimes they even met their boyfriends or life-partners online.

Since the Internet can facilitate both safe and unsafe sexual encounters, online HIV/STD prevention programs will continue to expand and develop and further research should be conducted to determine how best to facilitate a reduction in sexual risk. Additionally, traditional HIV/STD prevention programs must also find ways to address the specific prevention needs of men who meet sex partners online. Programs that emphasize and build on the Internet's strengths and assets, such as its exceptionally wide reach and the online environment's ability to foster self-empowerment, will be more meaningful to the target population of gay/bisexual men than those that only focus on epidemiological concerns.

14 Halflings and ogres and elves, oh my!

Sex, love, and relationships in EverQuest

Brandee Woleslagle

> The really cool thing that happened in this game is I found love again. I started playing this game because I had just gotten out of a nasty marriage . . . I would have never started a relationship in person. In this instance I fell in love before I knew it was happening.
>
> (April*, forty-one-year-old female, Kansas)

Many people would balk if you told them that your romantic partner is a troll who practices magic, slays dragons, and carries a wooden cudgel the size of her out-of-proportion head. Yet players of EverQuest**, a massively multiplayer online role-playing game (MMORPG), would probably just nod and ask how you met.

For several years Sony Online Entertainment dominated the MMORPG market with *EverQuest*, their best selling online game. Boasting 420,000 subscribers with more than 100,000 online at any one time, Sony has created a digital environment where players from around the globe log on to a three-dimensional fantasy world to play, socialize, and fight alongside one another.

For many, EverQuest is not a casual pastime. Participants rarely play less than two to three hours a day, a couple of days a week, while more serious gamers will play six to eight hours each weekday, with marathon stints of thirty or more hours over the weekend. Unsurprisingly, friendships form among players, which sometimes evolve into romantic partnerships.

It is important to understand the meaningfulness of relationships that are taking place in cyberspace. These relationships—which develop through chat programs, message boards, email, or in game environments—are becoming commonplace as more people gain access to the Internet. Yet when the topic of online romance is broached skeptics are still likely to say, "but it is not real!"

In order to gain an understanding of the relationships that are formed in online role-playing games, I conducted ethnographic research in the realm of EverQuest in late 2003. I held thirty-seven, in-depth interviews with participants ranging from age eighteen to sixty. The interviews were conducted online within the game world, allowing me to speak with individuals from five countries, and across the United States. Based on this study, I have found that relationships in EverQuest take several different forms.

---

*Names changed to protect privacy.
**EverQuest is a registered trademark of Sony Computer Entertainment America, Inc.

The consummate relationship

For some, a relationship that begins in the game blossoms into a full-fledged romance and a long-term relationship or marriage.

Kelly*, a twenty-six-year-old gamer from Pennsylvania, met her husband in the midst of a battle between blue-skinned orcs. While fighting alongside her, Kelly's husband-to-be made a comment that sparked her interest: he asked her if she wanted a kitten. Within one week she "just knew" that she had found her soul mate. A month after their in-game introduction, they decided to meet face-to-face.

Two years later, Kelly and Martin* married in two different ceremonies, one online and one offline. Kelly recalls that "it felt almost surreal because of that, like for some strange moment I really was my character. When we got married in real life, a bunch of our game friends who were at that (in-game) wedding were at the real wedding too."

Kelly and Martin's story is not atypical. During the course of my research I found that many people are meeting in EverQuest and taking their relationships offline. Shared interest in the game, and the ability to spend time with one another while playing, are some of the major forces behind these couplings. The amount of chatting generally multiplies after players exchange phone numbers and email addresses. The romance may culminate in a face-to-face meeting, which typically involves several days tucked away in a bedroom.

The online-only love affair

Not all romances end with the proverbial "happily ever after." There are those relationships that can never cross the digital boundary. Candace*, a nineteen-year-old female player from Ohio, is currently in a romantic partnership with John*, a married, fifty-two-year-old male.

Candace said of her relationship:

> I think we both understand that this is more of a fantasy relationship, since obviously it wouldn't work (offline), but we both wish it could be so much more. I think that kind of eats at both of us sometimes, but we're also not stupid, so we know what has to be.

Candace made it clear during the course of our interview that she was in love with John, and he with her. Candace added that "he's finally admitted that he's crossed the acceptable line in his feelings for me—I think if we lived closer together, there probably would have been a 'real' affair going on."

Candace and John ultimately decided not to take their relationship offline because both already have partners and too many miles between them. But other couples found other insurmountable obstacles, such as vast age differences. Common to these relationships are the intense feelings people have for one another, even if circumstances preclude them from taking the relationships offline.

The role-play relationship

A third type of relationship that occurs in *EverQuest* is based in role-play and does not involve attraction between the real-life partners. Instead, gamers initiate this type of relationship as "something to do" in addition to fighting monsters or tailoring tunics; role-playing a relationship adds to the atmosphere of the game.

Roxanne* described her role-play relationship as "mostly just a flirty fun relationship, kinda like the guy you flirt with just because it's a lot of fun, but you'd never really be serious about."

Adding role-play relationships to the game is a creative outlet for many people. In fact, players have created numerous websites and forums dedicated strictly to role-play, allowing players to share tales of their characters progression in the world of EverQuest outside of the game.

The cybersexual relationship

Finally, some relationships are purely for virtual sex. Sex on the Internet is no secret; perhaps less well known is the number of people who are finding sexual partners in the MMORPG environment. While cybersex occurs in all of the relationship types mentioned above, sex is the *raison d'être* for this partnership.

Perhaps the safest sex to be had, masturbating while chatting with another player is a common sexual activity. Veronica*, a sixty-year-old female player from Canada, uses some of her time while in game to find lovers. In order to find willing partners, Veronica sends private messages to players and hopes for a positive—and equally flirtatious—response.

Veronica said of her cyber relationships: "I am in total control here, I can disappear at any time, it is fun, a little dangerous, and it satisfies my (sexual) needs at this time."

Veronica is not alone in her quest for sexual partners. Matthew*, a thirty-three-year-old male from Illinois, has had many sexual relationships in the game:

> In this game I have met people of every sexual persuasion. I have met women who are hardcore dominatrixes and who think nothing of having their submissives make sounds like characters from the game, and I have met all manner of submissives and everything in between.

The cybersexual relationships experienced by these participants allow them to express their sexuality. While the participants often do not have long-lasting relationships, the time that they spend with their partners is intensely satisfying.

The future of researching online romances

EverQuest is not the only MMORPG where gamers are forming romances. Researchers interested in pursuing this topic further may find different relationship structures in past or future games or nonfantasy games such as City of Heroes with its comic book setting.

People enter digital worlds in order to have fun, play a game, or become a knight in shining armor. At the same time, people are forming lifelong commitments with partners as a result of meeting during the frivolity of game play. As Christine* put it, "it certainly is something to tell the kids. It definitely beats 'I met him in a bar!'"

15 *Finding Nemo* and transgender creatures

Judith Halberstam

In this short chapter I will explore the representation of transgenderism in popular culture. Using the framework of "natural diversity" adapted from a more recent stereotype in Joan Roughgarden's book, *Evolution's Rainbow*, I will read popular images of transgender beings (human and otherwise) as potential sources for the reconceptualization of binary gender. In her book, Roughgarden puts pressure on the Darwinian narrative of evolution by giving alternative interpretations of intermediate genders, cooperative behavior, and competitive struggle in the animal world. Arguing that researchers project narratives like "survival of the fittest" onto phenomena that could as easily be interpreted according to some other logic, Roughgarden allows us to see friendship systems between animals where other researchers have only seen competition; she replaces Darwin's theory of "sexual selection" with a concept of "social selection" and she rejects "the primacy of individualism" in favor of cooperative development. Roughgarden's interpretations of creatures that change sex, engage in same-sex erotics, or switch sex roles are refreshingly original and they reveal the extent to which contemporary theories of human cross-gender identification are limited by their commitment to dreary and unimaginative accounts of the body, the self, and diversity.

Popular culture produces, almost accidentally, plenty of narratives of belonging, relating, and evolving and they often associate these narratives with, or at least in proximity to, transgender characters. For example, an odd little animated film about a lost fish positioned queerness, and transgender queerness at that, in ways that may be helpful to us as we look for inspired conceptions of transgender difference. *Finding Nemo* told the story of a clownfish family that, in the film's tragic opening, is decimated by a hungry shark. The mother fish and almost all of her eggs are consumed, leaving a very anxious adult male fish, Marlin, with one slightly disabled offspring (he has a small fin on one side), Nemo. Marlin, whose voice is supplied by Albert Brooks, becomes understandably paranoid about the safety of his only son and he nervously, and even hysterically, tries to guard him from all of the dangers of the deep. Inevitably Nemo grows tired of his father's ministrations and, in a fit of oedipal rebellion, he tells his father he hates him and swims off recklessly into the open sea only to be netted by a diver and placed in a fish bowl in a dentist's office. Marlin, his paranoid fears now realized, begins a mad search for his missing son and swims his way to Sydney, Australia. When he finally finds him, he and Nemo orchestrate a fish uprising against their human jailors and they work out a different, non-oedipal, non-paranoid mode of relation.

Like *Chicken Run*, then, the Gramscian cartoon about organic chicken intellectuals— Gramscian in the sense that it understands revolutionary leaders as emerging from within the proletarian class itself—*Finding Nemo* weds its story of family to a tale of successful collective opposition to enslavement, forced labor, and commodification. And, like *Dude, Where's My Car* and *50 First Dates*, *Finding Nemo* exposes the limits to normal forms of knowledge and it casts forgetfulness as a powerful obstacle to capitalist and patriarchal modes of transmission. *Finding Nemo* also makes queer coalition, here represented by a seemingly helpful bluefish named Dory whose voice is supplied by the very queer Ellen Degeneres, into a major component of the quest for freedom and the attempts to reinvent kinship, identity, and collectivity. Dory accompanies Marlin on his quest for Nemo.

Dory, however, suffers from short-term memory loss and so only remembers intermittently why she and Marlin are swimming to Australia. Her odd sense of time introduces absurdity into an otherwise rather straight narrative and it scrambles all temporal interactions. When explaining her memory problem to Marlin, Dory says she thinks she must have inherited it from her family but, then again, she comments, she cannot remember her family so she is not sure how she came to be afflicted. In her lack of family memory, her exile in the present tense, her ephemeral sense of knowledge, and her continuous sense of a lack of context, Dory offers fascinating models of queer time (short-term memory), queer knowledge practices (ephemeral insights), and anti-familial kinship. In other words, she counters family time, with its long genealogical lines of transmission, with the time of the here and the now. The queerness of her lack of memory has to do with the way that she can never place herself in relation to others in terms of biogenetic kinship or lines of familial connection. By aiding Marlin without desiring him, finding Nemo without mothering him, and going on a journey without a goal, Dory offers us a model of cooperation that is not dependent upon payment or remunerative alliance. Dory, literally, swims alongside the broken family without becoming part of it and she helps to repair familial bonds without being invested in knowing specifically what the relations between Marlin and Nemo might be. The fact that they are father and son is of no more interest to her than if they were lovers or brothers, strangers or friends.

I focus here on *Finding Nemo* because I believe that popular culture, particularly non-earnest and non-serious popular culture, can offer narratives and images for the project of thinking through what J.K. Gibson-Graham calls "non-capitalist imaginaries." Furthermore, *Finding Nemo* covertly harbors a transgender narrative about transformation. Clownfish, we learn from Joan Roughgarden, are one of many species of fish that can, and often do, change sex. In *Evolution's Rainbow* Roughgarden writes that most biologists observe "nature" through a narrow and biased lens of socio-normativity and they, therefore, misinterpret all kinds of biodiversity. Transsexual fish, hermaphroditic hyenas, non-monogamous birds, homosexual lizards all play a role in the survival and evolution of the species, but mostly their function has been misunderstood and folded into rigid and unimaginative familial schemes of reproductive zeal and the survival of the fittest. Roughgarden explains that human observers misread competition into often cooperative activities, they misunderstand the relations between strength and dominance, and they overestimate the primacy of reproductive dynamics. In the case of the clownfish, according to Roughgarden, the mating couple does tend to be monogamous, so much so that if the female partner should perish (as she does in *Finding Nemo*), the male fish will transsex and become female. She will then mate with one of her offspring to recreate a kinship circuit. Roughgarden explains clownfish behavior, along with all kinds of other such morphing and shifting, less as evidence of the dominance of the reproductive circuit and more as an adaptive process of affiliation that creates stable community rather than familial structures.

Roughgarden's remarkable readings of biodiversity and "social," as opposed to "sexual," selection ask us to reconsider the very process of evolution as well as the nature and function of diversity. Dory, for example, in *Finding Nemo*, becomes recognizable in her relation to family if we use Roughgarden's narratives of social cooperation and the sharing of resources within any given animal community to replace hackneyed notions of the dominance of the biological family, the centrality and stability of the parent–child bonds, and the deliberate exclusion of non-relatives. And Marlin's overprotective parenting must now be read as a mode of transgender morphing in which he has changed from male to female. *Finding Nemo*, with its subtle critique of oedipal narratives of pleasure and danger, with its inspiring visions of collective fish rebellions, and with its queer models of friendship and affiliation, speaks directly to a queer feminist imagery and the possibilities of social change. In this film, as in a number of blockbuster films of the last few years, memory is linked in very material ways to the project of re-imagining kinship. *Finding Nemo* is just one of a spate of recent films (including *Dude, Where's My Car, 50 First Dates, Memento*) in which short-term memory loss plays a major role. In many of these films, transgender characters form the backdrop for the increasingly Byzantine methods by which heterosexual relations are cast as both inevitable and utterly scripted.

There is not time here to discuss in detail the significance of the "forgetful" films, but this developing genre does deserve some further thought, particularly since the drama of forgetfulness often plays out in relation to a host of transgender characters. In *Fifty First Dates*, for example, a film in which Drew Barrymore plays a woman afflicted by short-term memory loss due to an injury to her "temporal lobe" and Adam Sandler plays the man who tries to woo her, starting over every day, there are at least three transgender characters—the steroid addicted brother, the androgynous zoo-worker, and an old friend of Lucy's who has transformed from Jennifer to John—and also some animal subplots involving a randy penguin and a polyamorous but constipated walrus. The three transgender characters serve no obvious purpose in terms of advancing the narrative. Like the animals, they are supposed to represent the diversity of nature and culture! The transgender characters in both *Finding Nemo* and *50 First Dates* allow the films to project pathology away from the oddly sinister scenario of the romantic hero wooing the memory-deficient heroine everyday by reminding her of her place in the patriarchal family. The transgender characters symbolically represent the general disorder that has been created by disruptions to the family system. A conservative reading of such films might lead us to conclude that popular culture is remembering nostalgically a mythical time of continuity, locatedness, stability that is associated with the nuclear family and gender stability, that has to be energetically recreated in their absence.

The more hopeful reading of the genre and of the notion of gender and collectivity that it provokes might see the forgetful blue fish in *Finding Nemo* and the temporally challenged chick in *50 First Dates* as opportunities to think about the meaning of transgenderism in popular culture and the associations that popular culture unwittingly makes between social transformation and bodily change. The theme of forgetfulness links in interesting ways to transgender and particularly transsexual self-narratives because many TG and TS people have to "forget" their pasts as male or female in order to realize their adult genders. All of these films cast forgetfulness as an affliction associated with immaturity—adolescence even—and all recommend hetero marriage as a way of fixing, once and for all, the jarring sensation of waking up every day and not knowing who you are, where you have been, and where you are going. But I suggest that we recognize forgetting as a transgender trope and as a way of relieving the transgender subject from playing out his or her anatomy as destiny; *Finding Nemo*, surprisingly, with its emphasis on gender-morphing fish, forgetfulness, and non-familial affiliations constitutes a beautiful and inspiring allegory for transgender becoming.

16　*The L Word*

A little something for the femmetrosexual?

Kris Scott Martí

The L Word is Showtime's foray in lesbian and gay programming. It is the good—if bland—twin to the American version of the British series, *Queer As Folk*. Swooping over a dreamy and sensuous Los Angeles, *The L Word*'s action is set in a cozy west side neighborhood of craftsman-styled bungalows, where gay daddy groups walk—yes, I said *walk*—to their support groups and nary a strip mall is seen. The show opens with a new lesbian stereotype: Bette and Tina, a gorgeous mixed ethnicity couple, who are preparing to get pregnant. As one of the gay male characters explained, "The old joke was, 'What do lesbians bring to their second date? . . . A Uhaul.' Now, the joke is, 'What do lesbians bring on a second date? A turkey baster!'"

Next door is Tim, the neighborhood straight guy whose girlfriend Jenny is flying from the Midwest to live with him. We also meet the friends: Dana, a closeted tennis pro; the young player Shane; her bisexual admirer Alice who is working on a hardcopy version of the online networking service Friendster; the lascivious cafe owner Marina; and the mysterious musician Kit.

The characters spend a lot of time mulling over dyke drama in the local cafe—one full of women who look like they just finished a *Jane* magazine photo shoot. During the course of the two-hour premiere directed by *Go Fish* writer/director/producer Rose Troche, we find out that the perfect couple isn't so perfect, the straight girl isn't so straight, the closeted athlete is paying for remaining closeted, and lesbians in LA don't have pets or queer friends.

Commentary about *The L Word* has set some online lesbian bulletin boards ablaze with complaints of misrepresentation and non-representation of many real-life lesbians' concerns. Bulletin board writers also wonder whether images of lesbians should be used at all in the consumer oriented and often exploitive medium of TV.

The show, in some ways, is not about lesbians at all. Instead, it is about sensually stunning women in stylish outfits looking at and longing to have sex with whomever makes a more flattering accessory.

What we are witnessing on *The L Word* is the refinement of the "femmetrosexual"—where image is more important than content. Mark Simpson coined the term "metrosexual" to describe straight men who follow the fashion tastes of gay men. In *Salon* magazine, Simpson claimed to be a "lesbosexual," implying that being a lesbosexual is an *absence* of style—and, in turn, liberation from the time-consuming activities required to maintain the high style of the metrosexual. *The L Word* is the dressed up, well-heeled, and lipstick sporting epitome of metrosexuality for women.

The ladies of *The L Word* look like rock stars and live in Pottery Barn perfection. The "straight girl," Jenny, catches on to this reality right away; she dresses up for her dates with a woman but not for her man. Even the nurturing would-be mother Tina is thrown into a serious quandary—more in the style of an after school special than any serious introspection—about whether she wants to use an African American sperm donor. After sweating, hyperventilating, and generally acting like a 1950s television hausfrau, she finally justifies her hysterics to her partner. Tina doesn't want to disadvantage the child any more than necessary, and already the kid will have two mommies. The fact that her partner is African American and Caucasian suggests that these racial dynamics will be an ongoing issue for future episodes.

After the initial character development and conflicts, this luscious confection chock full of frontal nudity and brooding sexual confusion is fun to watch. *The L Word*'s premier was also interesting because it went beyond the stereotypical public imagination of what a lesbian is; instead *The L Word* investigates the not-so-fabulous world of average adulthood with all its loneliness, anxiety, betrayal, and defeat. As a lesbian, I enjoyed watching successful, well-dressed women ranting about the women they live with or want to love.

17 *Six Feet Under* brings abortion to the surface

Tracy A. Weitz and Anthony Hunter

Abortion is one of the most commonly performed medical procedures, but when was the last time you saw someone on TV have the procedure? Although there are over 1.3 million abortions ever year in the United States, abortion is rarely depicted in mainstream television. Whereas a decided majority of the US population is pro-choice, television content appears to represent the voice of the pro-life constituency. Even with the growth of cable programming, which flaunts the rejection of conservative network standards related to language, violence, and sexuality, abortion continues to be too controversial to present in any substantial way. Despite "politically correct" attempts to pay lip service to supporting a woman's right to choose, main female characters rarely go through with an abortion.

In the routine television storyline, a woman confronted with an unintended pregnancy considers all her options (abortion, adoption, or continuation with the pregnancy). Inevitably, she decides to have the child or, miraculously, she has a miscarriage. An example comes from the popular and award-winning series *Sex in the City*. As the show's official HBO Web site explained, Miranda Hobbes had planned on an abortion, but just before the procedure she changed her mind. Years earlier another "feminist character," Murphy Brown, decided that age and resources allowed her to have the child out-of-wedlock. Although she engendered Vice President Dan Quayle's ire, the network won support from abortion opposition groups who embraced Murphy's decision. Dawson's mother on *Dawson's Creek* was actually talked out of an abortion by her son, and Andrea on *Beverly Hills 90210* decided to continue her pregnancy and opt out of going to Yale University. In perhaps the most melodramatic storyline, Jo on *Melrose Place* chose to have her drug-dealing ex-boyfriend's baby, even though she was forced to kill the boyfriend to save her life. Although each of these women waxed poetically about supporting the right to choose, none of them actually chose to have an abortion.

For the women on TV who do not continue their unintended pregnancies, most often their pregnancies conveniently take care of themselves. Julia on *Party of Five* had a miscarriage before she was able to get to the abortion clinic. Amanda on *Melrose Place* had a ruptured ectopic pregnancy that would have left her sterile. Like their counterparts who continued their pregnancies, these characters "seriously" considered having an abortion. Such plot resolutions allow producers and network officials to stir interest around the topic of abortion without having to deal with the impact on the storyline should a character choose to have a child or an abortion. Critics on both sides can be mollified: pro-choice supporters can envision that the woman "would have gone through with it" and abortion opponents can argue that the character would have changed her mind.

Some characters have been bold enough to admit having had an abortion in the past. However, even a show like *Cagney and Lacey*—which had two female protagonists and was considered very progressive—could only have a lead character admit to having had an abortion within the context of choosing to continue a current pregnancy. A few other television programs have used an abortion storyline, including *Law and Order: Criminal Intent*, which covered the killing of an abortion provider, and *ER*, in which a onetime client has an abortion. *Everwood* included the story of a young girl who obtains an abortion from a doctor only after her main physician decides he can not provide her care. But only *Maude* in 1972 and *All My Children* in 1973 dared to have main characters who obtained abortions. That is, until now.

In May 2003 HBO bravely broke a long-established taboo by having Claire undergo an abortion on *Six Feet Under*. This action represents a positive first step toward addressing a common life experience for women. Despite this promising start, the storyline reverted to traditional pro-life messages in both its portrayal of abortion provision and in its comparison of a fetus with a fully developed baby.

Episode thirty-eight: abortion provision

In *Six Feet Under*'s thirty-eighth episode "Twilight" (directed by Kathy Bates and written by Craig Wright), Claire discovers that she is pregnant by her estranged boyfriend, Russell. The official HBO Web site summarizes the episode: "Claire makes a difficult choice as well: to terminate her pregnancy." The episode doesn't show Claire's decision-making process, but the nonchalant manner in which she asks Brenda for a ride to the clinic does not imply difficulty. "'Do you think you could give me a ride?' Claire asks. 'I have to get an abortion.'"[1] The Web site's description of the abortion decision as "difficult" foreshadows what is to come. In episode thirty-nine producers of the show seem to hedge their position on abortion by demonstrating Claire's conflicted feelings.

In this episode Claire undergoes an abortion according to the worst stereotypes about abortion provision. The impersonal and highly medical portrayal of the procedure demonstrates the extent to which the anti-choice rhetoric of abortion has become an accepted interpretation of reality. At the clinic Claire and Brenda sit in a waiting room surrounded by other women, devoid of any positive support. Claire is called from the waiting room with all the other women, en masse, and is shown in a room wearing a surgical gown undergoing what appears to be general anesthesia.

The viewer is led to believe that Claire's experience is routine for abortion. The episode's name "Twilight" stands for the type of anesthesia used for some abortion procedures. Abortion is portrayed as starkly medical and complicated, as well as grossly impersonal.

Postings on the *Six Feet Under* (SFU) Bulletin Board[2] demonstrate the extent to which this image took hold. One fan asked, "Do abortion clinics really function in such a factory like manner?"(simiulacra 5/18/03).

Others respond:

– The Abortions 'R Us place was like a factory. (isyou 5/18/03)
– [T]he way they called all the girl's names; like hearding (*sic*) animals (at the clinic). (KLV21 6/2/03)

- The writers on the show were treating abortion exactly like it is in real life . . . Abortion clinics do "cattle call" the patients in and it is usually an emotional hardship on the pregnant women. (Karen2240 6/2/03)
- YOU GOT THAT RIGHT! It is done in a "cattle call" fashion and it couldn't be any more accurate than that, as unfortunate as it may seem. (bajoros 6/2/03)
- The writers simply let it "all hang out," showing a typical clinic without comment or judgement (*sic*). If it's an eye opener to the audience, then good. (meridithc6/2/03)

Why not the "abortion pill?"

One of the hopes of the 2000 US approval of mifepristone (also known as the "abortion pill" or RU486 in France) was that abortion could be performed in regular healthcare providers' offices rather than in clinics, with minimal medical intervention. The negative imagery *Six Feet Under* fans portray in these bulletin board postings reflect the importance of continuing the effort to integrate abortion back into primary care, and to continue to move away from the idea that abortion is provided according to an impersonal clinic-based model.

With that said, it is also important to acknowledge that most abortion clinics do not operate in such a manner. Instead, the majority of early abortions are performed under local anesthesia while a patient wears her own clothes rather than a surgical gown. Women are also given individualized, personal, and compassionate care. Research on the quality of abortion care has demonstrated overwhelmingly high satisfaction among abortion clients.[3] The dialogue between the *Six Feet Under* fans exposes the extent to which anti-abortion perspectives have become the accepted interpretation. The fan dialogue about *Six Feet Under* also exposes the damage done by television's failure to realistically portray abortion provision.

That *Six Feet Under* does not include medical abortion is disappointing. Rather than reinforcing old stereotypes, the writers and producers could have explored new ground. They could have educated the public about medical abortion while also providing entertaining television. The confusion and lack of knowledge about medical abortion is apparent in the following exchange[4] among *Six Feet Under* fans:

- These days, many early pregnancies are ended with RU486. Are the prolifers picketing drugstores these days? (sandgann 5/19/03).
- RU486 isn't available at the drugstore, either. You have to get it at a clinic, and you have to get it the very next morning. (titannia 5/19/03)
- You're thinking of the morning-after pill. That's different from RU-486. (wolfgirl 6/4/03)
- You can only get the abortion pill at an abortion clinic, and you have to (be) watched while it takes effect. (Maggiespancake 5/19/03)

Episode thirty-nine: a fetus becomes a baby in the "afterlife"

The greatest disappointment of *Six Feet Under*'s groundbreaking abortion story is its attempt to balance appeals from both pro-choice and pro-life viewers. Whereas episode thirty-eight shows Claire having an abortion without ramifications, episode thirty-nine ("I'm Sorry, I'm Lost," directed by Alan Ball and written by Jill Solway) appeases those who might have opposed her decision. The HBO official Web site describes this episode:

"Claire remains conflicted over the abortion." During the episode her dead father takes her on a visit to the afterlife where she "encounters beatific versions of people she's cared for and lost: Lisa, Gabe Dimas—and the baby she decided not to have."[5] During her exchange with Lisa, Claire is asked to care for Lisa's living child in exchange for Lisa caring for the "baby" Claire aborted. As one fan noted: "What makes me wonder about the Lisa/Claire exchange is why they used a full-term baby as Claire's baby and everyone else in the 'afterlife' were exactly the age they were when they died." (mpasq 6/2/03).[6]

Again, postings to the *Six Feet Under* fans bulletin board demonstrate the limitations of the approach and its direct appeal to those who oppose abortion:

– Although I do not identify myself in the pro-life (or anti-abortion) camp, I cannot interpret the image of Claire seeing her aborted baby with Lisa in the afterlife as anything but a pro-life statement. (russjourn 6/1/03)
– Yet they had her have the abortion in the first place? I think the writers did a great job of trying to please everyone. The pro-choicers for letting her decide to have the abortion and the pro-lifers for giving the baby such a peaceful place of rest. (NakkisGirl 6/1/03)
– I did think it was strange that the guy who wrote "twilight" said that SFU would be taking a no opinion stance on the abortion thing. [The heaven] scene made a definite statement. (1heather247 6/1/03)

What is clear from this exchange is how directly the fans understand the storyline to be part of a larger public dialogue about abortion.

The power of television

Six Feet Under should be commended for its courage to have a primary character choose an abortion. At the same time, however, the show reinforces old images of abortion provision and makes an overt appeal to abortion opponents. Criticism of the coverage of abortion on *Six Feet Under* should not discourage other shows from taking the bold step to have main characters choose to have abortions when faced with unintended pregnancies. Rather, the limitations explored in this review should serve as appeals to writers and producers to forge ahead and explore new ground, rather than to find compromises between the "pro-choice" and the "pro-life" positions. Abortion remains fiercely polemic and therefore appeals as a plotline for courageous television.

Television, however, can be used as a force in changing the way we feel about issues. Thirty years ago a positive storyline about a gay character would have seemed impossible. Today, however, shows such as *Six Feet Under, Will and Grace, Ellen* and *The L Word* have unapologetically presented gay characters. In these shows the related storylines have moved beyond the question of whether such lifestyle choices are wrong and immoral to a richer discussion on what it is to be gay in the world. These characters are allowed to have full lives and relationships, and to integrate being gay with other aspects of the plot.

Only by presenting abortion as what it is—a commonplace reality—can the media move away from conventional stories and begin to reflect the complexity and individuality of women's experiences. Women should be allowed to have abortions and talk about them, without blatant attempts to pacify those who oppose abortion. HBO's tentative first step should not be the last one.

Notes

1   HBO. *Six Feet Under*: Episode 38 "Twilight". Home Box Office. Available at: http://www.hbo.com/sixfeetunder/episode/season3/sea3_eps12.shtml. Accessed July 29, 2003.
2   HBO *Six Feet Under* Bulletin Boards. Available at: http://boards.hbo.com/forum.jsp?forum=117. Accessed July 29, 2003.
3   The Picker Institute. 1999. *The Patient's Perspective: Quality of Abortion Care*. Menlo Park, CA: Kaiser Family Foundation.
4   HBO *Six Feet Under* Bulletin Boards. Available at: http://boards.hbo.com/forum.jsp?forum=117. Accessed July 29, 2003.
5   HBO. *Six Feet Under*: Episode 39 "I'm Sorry, I'm Lost". Home Box Office. Available at: http://www.hbo.com/sixfeetunder/episode/season3/sea3_eps13.shtml. Accessed July 29, 2003.
6   HBO *Six Feet Under* Bulletin Boards. Available at: http://boards.hbo.com/forum.jsp?forum=117. Accessed July 29, 2003.

18 The pornography of consumption/ the consumption of pornography

Linda Williams

It is an industry in which quantity typically trumps quality—an industry that gluts the market with goods of questionable social value. The captains are not selling burgers. They are selling sex.

Where Hollywood makes approximately four hundred films a year, the porn industry makes ten to eleven thousand a year and there are 700 million porn rentals annually. Yearly pornography revenues—which in one estimation include magazines, Internet websites, cable, in-room hotel movies, and sex toys—total between $10 to $50 billion.

And yet, pornography is a very different kind of excess. Unlike the rise of fast food, the "McDonaldization" of porn marks an important shift in the place of sexuality in our contemporary American culture. Of course, much pornography does offer predictable representations of heterosexual male fantasies, but this is just one direction of a genre that can also give us decidedly unglamorous San Francisco lesbians having sex with dildos on cluttered kitchen tables. Sometimes pornography can verge toward . . . something.

The pornography of consumption

Social critics have mobilized a previously existing distaste for the sheer lowness of pornography to drive home important arguments about the loss of the real and the emptiness of contemporary consumption. As George Ritzer—author of *The McDonaldization of Society* and *The Globalization of Nothing*—puts it, pornography stands for the obscenity of a consumption that lacks substantive content. In other words, pornography represents the wasteful, greedy, and immoral consumption of "nothing."

This "pornography of consumption" is a rhetorically powerful way to describe the excess of our contemporary consumer society. This society superficially sates itself on useless "goods" whose only real function is to lead to the consumption of more goods, none of which really satisfies in any deep or lasting way.

The metaphor seems apt because of pornography's sheer lowness on the scale of cultural values. If ever there was a cultural "good" or product that was without what sociologist Pierre Bourdieu calls "distinction," then moving image pornography is it. It is vulgar, it is low. It may help sexually hungry people sate sexual desires late at night in an anonymous hotel room, but it does not deeply satisfy. It is, of all consumer goods available in American culture, the one we can all most easily agree to hate.

The metaphor of a pornography of consumption also seems befitting because pornography connotes the pervasive sexualization—and, by extension, feminization— of this culture. Hardly anything in contemporary consumer culture is sold without the aid of a typically feminine "sex appeal." French sociologist Jean Baudrillard writes, "sexuality is 'at the forefront' of consumer society, spectacularly over-determining the entire signifying field of mass communications."

Finally, the metaphor seems suitable because pornography not only shows sex but makes sex hypervisible. Cars are photographed in television advertising, much the way bodies in moving-image pornography or weapons in CNN inserts are photographed: from every possible angle. Film critic Richard Dyer calls the extreme close-up shots "plumbing shots." John Waters has remarked that porn always looks to him "like open-heart surgery."

But while there is a pornograph*ic* nature of American consumption practices, pornography—as in moving images of explicit sex—is not itself pornograph*ic*. Pornography deserves a better, more precise, critique than that leveled against the generic, uprooted, dehumanized, immoral, nothingness of McDonald's or McMansions.

From obscene to on/scene

Pornography as a genre has existed since the rise of mass media—print, lithography, photograph, film and video. If we look at its history, however, we see that it is only in the last thirty years that it has been available, in the form of moving images, to large numbers of the public.

Recently, the details about explicit sex acts performed by politicians, celebrities, and porn stars have become increasingly familiar to average people. This is not to say that sexually explicit representation is without controversy or embarrassment. We have certainly not attained the "end of obscenity" once optimistically predicted in the late 1960s by Charles Rembar. It is to say, however, that long before it surfaced as news from the oval office, a contemporary "speaking sex" had ceased to be a private bedroom-only matter and had come, as I like to put it, "on/scene."

The term on/scene suggests that to think of pornography as obscene is, today, something of an anachronism. The ultimate reason for this has less to do with obscenity law than with the remarkable transition discourses of sexuality have made from shameful whispers to a key factor in the articulation of human identity itself. The incitement to speak and confess sexual secrets has been growing, according to historian Michel Foucault, at least since the sixteenth century. Beginning in the twentieth century, and especially with Freud, however, sexual confession, of which the genre of pornography is most emphatically a form, has become central to who we think we are as individuals. For better or for worse, one effect of the explosion of discourses of sexuality has been a democratization of explicit sexual representations no longer cordoned off for specially entitled viewers.

Sexual representations whose very purpose is to arouse readers or viewers were once deemed ob/scene in the literal sense of being kept off—or "ob"—the public sphere have today insistently appeared in the new public/private realms of Internet and home video. I coined the term on/scenities to describe the paradoxical gesture by which American culture brings onto its public arena the very organs, acts, bodies, and pleasures that have heretofore been designated ob/scene and kept locked up for only a few. On/scenity marks the controversy and scandal of the increasingly public representations of diverse forms of sexuality and the fact that they have become increasingly available and quasi-normal.

So what does this on/scenity mean? Is it, on the level of sexual representation, the same thing as the democratization of dining out made possible by the standardization of fast foods? Certainly, there is much that is cheap, badly acted, and boringly repetitive about the genre. But some pornography differs from a Big Mac. Sometimes it can resist this predictability and become . . . something.

Equalizing sexualities

Pornography has been a crucial way in which emerging sexual minorities—either invisible or ridiculed in more mainstream representations—have recognized themselves as sexual beings on screen. The genre of moving image pornography, unlike the genre of fast food, can thus be seen as one of the ways in which American culture has been talking to itself about what constitutes "good"—arousing, hot, desirable—sex.

For example, in the early 1970s right alongside feature-length theatrical pornography like *Deep Throat* or *Behind the Green Door*, a parallel production and exhibition of titles like *Boys in the Sand* and *Sex Garage* graced the screens of emerging urban, gay neighborhoods. For the first time, emerging gay audiences were seeing and recognizing themselves on screen.

Even as silly a movie as the 1972 *Deep Throat* was talking to itself about new vociferous demands made by women for orgasm equity. The film's narrative solution of placing a clitoris in Linda Lovelace's throat was not satisfying to most women viewers but the resulting privileging of fellatio and "money shots"—external ejaculation in proximity to the woman's face—became a major trope of hardcore pornography that was no longer satisfied by the mere spectacle of penetration.

Unlike the sameness of most other standardized consumer products, pornography offers a surprising variety. Consider award-winning *Shock*, about the sexual fantasies of a patient in a laboratory undergoing shock treatment by a decidedly sadomasochistic female doctor. The protagonist, who seems to be a man but turns out to be woman, leads a chorus in a song about the deceitfulness of appearances. It is glossy, high-tech, and overproduced, a kind of *Matrix* avant la lettre. But it is also fascinating, even endearing, in its philosophical and aesthetic ambitions.

At the other end of the aesthetic spectrum is crudely shot and amateurishly acted dyke porn with primitive production qualities that contribute to the authentic nature of the sex acts and counter standard images of so-called lesbian sex in heterosexual videos. Indeed, all forms of pornography tending toward the amateur end of the spectrum are likely to deliver "something" because of their valuation of authenticity over glamour (no breast jobs allowed). These videos tend toward the *unique* and *local*. At the most amateurish end they consist of a single shot from a camera posed on a tripod. Debra and Earl from California, for example, "request correspondence from anyone viewing their tape." The tape is available in exchange for one showing the requestor's own sexual activity. Thus, the tape may only exist in a single copy, the very opposite of standardization of its industrial counterparts and, more or less, outside the capitalist economy all together. To further invoke Ritzer's terms, it is also specific to the *time* and *place* it is made (the actual California living room or bedroom of the couple), and it is *humanized* (Debra and Earl are themselves and they communicate together about what pleases them) and *enchanted* (certainly for them and they hope for someone else). There is nothing in the genre of franchised food that can offer such a genuinely oppositional resistance to standardization while still delivering a genre.

The list of humanized and enchanted pornographies can be extended beyond gay, lesbian, and amateur pornographies to videos of transsexual, s/m, bondage, amputees, geriatric, fat, ethnic, interracial, gonzo, and beyond.

The point should be clear: if you have seen and tasted a Big Mac, you may very well have seen and tasted them all. But if you have seen one pornographic feature you have emphatically *not* seen them all. Like Westerns, musicals, and films noir, pornography has remarkable deviations within the requisite standardization. And like these more respected Hollywood genres marketed on the basis of generic expectation, authors known for their distinctive styles within the confines of the pornography have emerged. In a genre that forty years ago never had a single name attached, we now see a proliferation of names: Radley Metzger, John Leslie, Michael Ninn, John Stagliano, Candida Royalle, and Jenna Jameson. McDonald's does not similarly celebrate its chefs.

Selling sexual fantasies is not the same thing as selling hamburgers. In critiquing America's overconsumption, we can reasonably say, as Ritzer implies, that the perversion for a small portion of the world's population to drive gas-guzzling cars forces other motorists to buy similar cars for self-protection. This is a perversion of need that is, in actual fact, immoral, and excessive.

To brand pornography with the same accusation is questionable because pornography's perversions are actually quite natural—built into the very structure of sexual desire and pleasure. Unless we wish to buy into an archaic productivist notion of sexuality as properly serving only reproductive ends, we cannot say the same thing of the proliferating perversions of contemporary pornography that we do of McMansions. Perversion of sexual instincts—in the literal sense of swerving away from "normal" sexual object (say, a man for a man rather than a man for a woman) or "normal" sexual aim (say exhibitionist ejaculation for all to see rather than vaginal intromission)—is not necessarily similarly immoral and is inherent to the work of sexuality itself. For sex is, as Freud put it, the most "unruly of the instincts," one that perpetually veers off from direct satisfaction to more circuitous routes. These unruly instincts are inherently perverse. Freud wrote, "No healthy person . . . can fail to make some addition [to sex] that might be called perverse to the normal sexual aim." Insofar as we do not proceed directly to heterosexual vaginal penetration with intromission, we, and the pornographies we may watch, are literarily perverted.

The consumption of pornography, then, is not, as Ritzer argues of the consumption of Big Macs, the consumption of nothing. "Nothing" to Ritzer is generic, lacking local context, lacking specific time, dehumanized, and disenchanted. Some pornography is unique, embedded in a specific time and place, humanized and (perhaps) even enchanted. But unlike a really good restaurant, pornography is not produced, as it once was, only for the elite. No longer the province of upper-class men, or as it later became, all men, it is now available to men, women, and sexual minorities who until the last ten years did not have a pornography of their own. In setting up the nothing/something continuum, Ritzer may be idealizing and nostalgicizing a time before industrialization, standardization, and democratization.

19 InnovAsian in pornography?

Asian American masculinity and the "porno revolution"

Amy Sueyoshi

U.C. Davis Professor Darrell Hamamoto declared in a 2003 *Salon* article that Asian Americans needed "sexual healing" and he, as the "doctor," had arrived.

Hamamoto had just filmed *Skin on Skin*, a fifty-minute porn that hoped to reclaim Asian American male sexuality from castration in American media. America had brutally emasculated Asian men, rendering them sexually undesirable even to their "yella womenz," explained Hamamoto. By casting an Asian American man to play the sexual partner of an Asian American woman, he saw his project as an innovative way to fight the damaging effects of colonialism and racism upon Asian American sexuality.

Rallying around the unjust emasculation of Asian American men has long appeared to be cause célèbre among those engaged in Asian American issues. From Fu Manchu in the 1930s to *Sixteen Candles'* Long Duk Dong in the 1980s, depictions of Asian American men have appeared less than "manly" in popular culture.

James Hou, a filmmaker and former student of Hamamoto's, traced the making of *Skin on Skin* in a documentary titled *Masters of the Pillow*. More so than *Skin on Skin* itself, Hou's documentary powerfully drew media attention to Hamamoto's porn project. Between February 2003 and November 2004 over twenty articles appeared in city dailies and online publications as a variety of film festivals screened the documentary. Newspapers such as the *Sacramento Bee* and the *Honolulu Star* jumped on Hamamoto's *Skin on Skin*. Comedy Central's *Daily Show* and NBC's *Tonight Show* both featured segments on the professor turned porn producer. Hamamoto himself declared a "porno revolution."

Hamamoto's work would ultimately prove more rote than radical, though. Not only would the porn itself appear numbingly mundane. Specific strains in gay porn had more powerfully resurrected Asian American male sexuality nearly a decade before *Skin on Skin*. Hamamoto took credit for a revolution already under way.

Hamamoto had indeed hoped to reassert the Asian male as more sexually potent, but the content of his porn would ultimately prove more successful at reinforcing images of Asian American women, rather than at re-imagining Asian American masculinity. A camera sequence that focused on the naked woman and her acts to service the man perpetuated stereotypes of Asian American women more than it salvaged the sexuality of Asian American men. Hamamoto's piece resembled the thousands of low-budget productions that fill the shelves of adult video stores throughout Asia.

Yet Hamamoto asserted that according to the emails he received, 99 percent of his "Asian American peeps" appreciated his innovation. Still, on one message board discussing his work at ModelMinority.com, a Web site dedicated to Asian American empowerment, reactions appeared less supportive. Out of sixteen different login IDs that contributed to an exchange of thirty-five comments, only nine appeared explicitly supportive. Four openly criticized Hamamoto's endeavor and three remained skeptical about the positive value of his work. For this online community dedicated to social justice for Asian Americans, support for *Skin on Skin* as a worthy endeavor appeared ambivalent.

Meanwhile, gay porn may have already more successfully reclaimed Asian American masculinity along Hamamoto's standards of ideal masculinity. Though filmmaker Richard Fung had pointed to the gay porn industry's history of racism in casting Asians as mere receptacles of sex, in the years that followed his seminal 1991 essay "Looking for my Penis," Asian American men appeared to be gaining significant sexual ground.

The gay porn production company Catalina Video, in particular, has produced close to twenty videos with Asian content catering to Asian Americans since the 1990s— significant considering Asian Americans make up about 5 percent of the US population, among which less than 10 percent are queer. While many certainly deployed "Oriental" clichés in titles and set decor, sexual interactions demonstrated the powerful sexuality of Asian American men. Muscled Asian Americans with impressive phalluses played confident "tops." *Asian Men Do* featured the handsome Tony Chan, six feet tall with a seven and a half inch penis. In *Fortune Nookie* when a penniless Asian American Brandon Lee faced lawyer fees to white attorney Jacob Scott, he offered sex in exchange. Notably, Jacob became the "bossy bottom" in anal sex.

Catalina Video promoted these Asian American actors with the language of unabashed "masculinity." A summary of *Asian Persuasion* described Brandon Lee's "thick meat." In *Crème of Sum Yung Gai* as well, when actor Al Wong penetrated fellow Asian American actor Dematthew Yung, Catalina wrote of Al sending in the "heavy artillery." Moreover, Catalina Video described its Far East Feature Series as showcasing "horny Asian studs getting man-nasty with their pals." The production company promoted their Asian actors as virile, sexual agents.

Gay porn star Brandon Lee may have been the true "pioneer" rather than Hamamoto. With an eight and a half-inch phallus, rounded muscles of a water polo player, and boyish good looks, the unrelenting top arrived in the porn industry seven years before the U.C. Davis academic. He dominated Catalina Video's Far East Features and cut across genres to their non-racialized Blockbuster series as an "Asian stud."

Might Hamamoto team up with Brandon Lee to reclaim Asian American male sexuality? Likely not. At the Visual Communications Film Festival in May 2004, co-producer of *Skin on Skin* and Hamamoto's girlfriend Funie Hsu posed their porn project as significant precisely because of its heterosexual context, battling against portrayals of Asian American men as effeminate and homosexual. Ironically, in the Asian American porn of Catalina Video, "gay" more likely signaled the type of masculinity that Hamamoto and Hsu coveted, rather than the effeminacy they loathed. Indeed, Asian gay masculinity might be the cure to the Asian straight man's gender woes.

Queer masculinities have been revolutionizing Asian American male sexuality, through not just production companies such as Catalina Video, but also independent transgender porn producers such as Christopher Lee. Because men of color have been denied access to normative (white) masculinity, creating alternative erotic ideals that incorporated existing realities of Asian American men were more compelling for many. While cultural critic Nguyen Tan Hoang would see Brandon Lee as reinforcing white mainstream models of ideal masculinity, Christopher Lee's erotic images more potently depart from the norm.

Yet, why are effeminate men necessarily considered undesirable? Why does sexuality have to play such a central role in our self-worth? Why do we need Asian American men in pornography? Indeed, the gender and sexual standards that we uncritically accept might prove to be the more powerful obstacle against socio-sexual justice. Scrutinizing these foundational issues might eventually lead more quickly down the path of "sexual healing" rather than any porn project. After all, the master's tools will likely never dismantle the master's house.

20 The Yin and Yang of sex work

Female and male prostitution
compared

Ann M. Lucas

Say the word "prostitute" and what comes to mind? A woman in revealing clothing standing atop four-inch platform shoes, soliciting prospective customers at night on the street, as johns cruise slowly by in their cars; she works for an exploitative pimp, or if not, she sells herself to feed the demands of her crack pipe or dime bag of heroin.

Despite a wealth of articles and books, both popular and scholarly, written on the topic of prostitution, the practice remains shrouded in stereotype. While it is true that the "typical" American prostitute is female, there is also a market for male sex workers. Female prostitutes, though, receive greater media scrutiny, social opprobrium, and police attention than male prostitutes, not only because of their greater numbers and visibility, but also because society has a strong interest in deterring female prostitution in order to shore up dominant norms about "good" (monogamous, modest, and noncommercial) female sexuality. Male prostitutes are not free of disapproval and arrest, but their prostitution activity is not the primary cause of such negative attention; rather, they stand at the intersection of social concerns about female prostitution and male homosexuality and, therefore, suffer indirectly from moral campaigns directed at these larger targets.

Who they are, who their customers are

The exact numbers of prostitutes, female or male, are impossible to obtain. Prostitution is illegal in every state, except for a few rural counties in Nevada that have legal brothels. Therefore, most prostitutes feel the need to conceal what they do in order to avoid arrest and social stigma.

According to estimates on female prostitution, street prostitutes comprise about 10 to 20 percent of the prostitution population nationwide, and perhaps about 30 percent in some cities, such as San Francisco, where the climate is more temperate year round. That means the large majority of female prostitutes are less visible to the public; 70 to 90 percent work indoors, in massage parlors, lingerie shops, strip clubs, illegal brothels, and the like, or in hotel rooms, private residences, and other private settings as escorts and call girls. Male prostitutes also work on the streets, in bars and clubs, and as escorts and call boys. Both male prostitutes of all types and indoor female prostitutes receive less media attention and scholarly study than street prostitutes, reinforcing our incorrect stereotypes.

Of female street prostitutes, figures from the late 1980s suggested that about 40 percent worked independently and 60 percent had pimps, although even fewer prostitutes may work with pimps today. But these figures become even shakier because the term "pimp" can be narrowly or broadly defined. That is, if a prostitute turns over any portion of her earnings to another, is she working for a pimp? What if he is her boyfriend who watches out for her while she solicits on the street? What if that person is her adult child or a roommate she supports while that person is unemployed or going through rehab? Some observers have argued that the "pimp" label is too widely applied by some researchers to any person who is supported with the earnings of prostitution. The term pimp, they say, should be reserved for those who engage in coercive or exploitative relationships with prostitutes and function as managers of a "stable" of women. Whatever its real incidence, true pimping is probably less common among male prostitutes than female prostitutes. Because male prostitutes are less commonly arrested, because they are less likely to be targeted by sexual predators, and because they tend to be better able to defend themselves physically, they are not as vulnerable to coercion from pimps. Female prostitutes, on the other hand, may need pimps for physical and legal protection.

The overwhelming majority of customers of both female and male prostitutes are men, although the number of women who hire prostitutes may be slowly rising. At some Caribbean resort destinations, female tourists hire local men as sexual companions; they are sometimes called "rent-a-dreads" in reference to the dreadlocks worn by many Jamaican men. In the United States the few women who do patronize prostitutes are usually accompanying a boyfriend or husband, rather than hiring a prostitute alone.

Although most customers are men, that does not say anything about the sexual preferences of prostitutes themselves. Certainly, sexual orientation affects their experiences with, and attitudes toward, customers. Straight women, lesbians, and bisexual women work as prostitutes serving male customers, just as straight, gay, and bisexual men work as prostitutes serving male customers. Transgendered women also work as prostitutes serving male customers.

Because the customer sees the prostitution transaction in sexual rather than economic terms, his actual sexual orientation is likely reflected in his choice of prostitutes, although his avowed sexual orientation may be different. That is, most men who hire a male prostitute enjoy or are curious about same-sex sexual activity, regardless of how they label themselves, and most men who hire female prostitutes enjoy opposite-sex sexual activity, even if they are not exclusively heterosexual. The same cannot be said about the sexualities of the individuals being paid.

The policing of prostitution

Law enforcement activity related to prostitution is not evenly distributed among prostitutes and customers, nor among types of prostitutes. Although street prostitutes are a minority of all prostitutes, they make up as much as 85 to 90 percent of prostitutes arrested. Women of color who work on the streets are especially (and disproportionately) likely to draw police attention. According to estimates, women of color represent 40 to 45 percent of street prostitutes but 55 percent of those arrested and 85 percent of those given jail time. In other words, the racial, gender, and class inequities we see in the larger society are reflected in prostitution. Those already marginalized or disadvantaged in some fashion tend to pay the most for their transgressions.

Although there are more customers than prostitutes in the general population—most prostitutes could not earn a living otherwise—prostitution-related arrests overwhelmingly involve the service provider, not the customer. Prostitutes make up 80 to 90 percent of the arrests, with customers constituting the other 10 to 20 percent. Of all prostitution-related arrests, 60 to 70 percent are women (almost all of these women are prostitutes, with very few madams also arrested). Although some might claim the prostitute/customer arrest disparity is a valid policy decision since prostitutes are repeat offenders and, therefore, deserve more police attention, many patrons are also repeat customers. Absent the demand—it is estimated that there are five to eight customers on the streets for every prostitute working there—supply would diminish significantly.

Better explanations for the disparity are that many police officers share a general social belief that it is more morally offensive for women to sell sexual services than for men to purchase them—a "men are dogs" (but women are supposed to be pure) mentality. Moreover, many officers recognize that an arrest for soliciting prostitution will likely be more damaging to the customer, who may otherwise have a reputation as a respectable and law-abiding citizen, than for the prostitute for whom an arrest may simply be the cost of doing business. If the customer "can't help it" and has more to lose from an arrest, arresting the prostitute seems the better choice.

However, since it takes two people (or more) for the offense of prostitution to be committed, this disproportionate enforcement pattern is not justifiable. Certainly in some cities at specific times, there have been attempts to reverse this pattern by focusing enforcement activity on customers, particularly through the use of a variety of shaming tactics, from publishing the names of "johns" on television, in newspapers, on websites, on recorded messages, or on billboards, to vehicle impoundment and "John Schools." Still, these experiments have yet to revolutionize the policing of prostitution offenses in the United States.

The disparity between female prostitute arrests and male prostitute arrests may well reflect their proportions of the prostitute population, but that is not the entire explanation. It can be argued that police officers—who even today are mostly men—are largely uncomfortable posing undercover as potential patrons of male hustlers. As one male prostitute I interviewed put it, "Police will crack down on women before men, because . . . homophobia acts as . . . some protection for male [prostitutes]." In addition, the social outcry over male prostitution is minimal compared to that surrounding female prostitution, and thus citizens are less compelled to demand something be done to reduce this activity.

Stereotypes and arrest patterns reveal that the social stigma surrounding prostitution is not evenly distributed among all its participants. Rather, female prostitutes bear the brunt of social stigma, while male customers, although certainly not admired, largely escape the fear and loathing—not to mention harassment and attack—directed at prostitutes. Those critical of customers often find the men's behavior slightly odious but generally also believe that "boys will be boys."

A demand for male bodies

When prostitution is discussed as a social problem, it often is considered a phenomenon solely involving female service providers. Male prostitutes are invisible and neither "gigolos" nor male hustlers garner much attention. Although male prostitutes do receive their share of stigma in some situations, only a portion of it is based on prostitution. That is, among the general public, those most opposed to male prostitution are opposed to men having sex with men (paid or unpaid) in general. The objection to male prostitution is an artifact of the stigmatization of homosexuality. On the other hand, most of those opposed to female prostitution are particularly concerned about the commercial aspect of the transaction.

Still, some members of gay communities do stigmatize gay male prostitutes, objecting to the commercialization or commodification of sexuality and the negative image male prostitution brings to the larger gay population. This stigma, though, is not identical to that experienced by female prostitutes, either in form or intensity. Male prostitution does not have the same image of abuse and exploitation as female prostitution does, so it does not attract the same kinds of objections. In addition, a significant number of gay men, particularly urban gay men, see gay hustling as an adolescent rite of passage or youthful oat-sowing, rather than a practice that threatens "healthy" gay sexuality and relationships.

The future

The most humane approach to prostitution would be the decriminalization of consensual adult prostitution. This approach would enable those who choose to work as prostitutes, or to hire them, to escape the social stigma attached to prostitution. It would free up resources so that law enforcement could focus on more serious crimes. It would allow our society to discuss prostitution more fully and honestly, both in regard to its actual or potential benefits and its disadvantages. It would promote norms of professionalism within the industry. Without criminal status and a marginal social position, prostitutes who are victims of violent customers, abusive pimps, international traffickers, and the like, would be more likely to seek help. Decriminalization of prostitution would also promote greater social acceptance of sexual diversity in human societies.

Yet in the current political climate decriminalization of prostitution is highly unlikely. Indeed, compared to legalization (i.e., regulation), decriminalization might be unlikely in any context. As New York University law Professor Sylvia Law has argued, given that work, in general, is extensively regulated in our society, it is unreasonable to think that a practice as controversial as prostitution could escape regulation if it were no longer illegal. Should legalization ever be pursued as an alternative to criminalization, it ought to be designed with the participation of prostitutes and with prostitute welfare in mind, rather than as a way to raise revenue through taxes (a "government as pimp" approach), or a way to control a "dangerous" group through registration, fingerprinting, and disease testing. These latter approaches would simply replicate the abuses that occur under criminalization, and thus cannot truly constitute "reform."

21 Strip clubs and their regulars

Katherine Frank

Sexual services and products have long been a part of the US entertainment and leisure industries. In a 1997 article for *US News & World Report*, Eric Schlosser reported that in the prior year Americans spent "more than $8 billion on hard-core videos, peep shows, live sex acts, adult cable programming, sexual devices, computer porn, and sex magazines." The number of major strip clubs catering to heterosexually identified men nearly doubled between 1987 and 1992, and an estimate for late 1998 put the number of clubs at around 3,000 with annual revenues ranging from $500,000 to more than $5 million.

While some men dislike strip clubs or find them boring, a significant population of heterosexual American males are willing to spend their money on the kind of public, voyeuristic (although interactive) fantasy available in a no-contact strip club. Despite popular beliefs to the contrary, strippers are generally not selling sex to their customers in this type of club—although they are selling sexualized and gendered services. Rather than fulfilling a biological need for sexual release, as some pop sociobiological accounts suggest, or serving a masculine need for domination, strip clubs provide a kind of intermediate space (not work and not home, although related to both) in which men can experience their bodies and identities in particular pleasurable ways. In my book *G-Strings and Sympathy: Strip Club Regulars and Male Desire*, published in 2002, I investigated the sources and forms of men's pleasure. I demonstrated how the material inequalities and everyday lives of customers are intertwined with the meanings that customers attribute to their visits to strip clubs. While I cannot discuss all of the complexities underlying the men's motivations for their visits in this chapter, I suggest a few important aspects.

Strip clubs are stratified in terms of luxury, status, and other distinguishing features. Whereas strip clubs were once primarily located in "red light" areas of towns and cities associated with crime and prostitution, the upscale clubs are, now, quite often visible and they work to develop reputations for safety, comfort, and classiness. Drawing on cultural markers of status—such as luxury liquors, fine dining, valet parking, and private conference rooms—upscale clubs advertise themselves as places for businessmen to entertain clients or for middle-class professionals to visit after work. Dancers may be advertised as refined, well-educated women. Sophisticated sound and lighting equipment, multiple stages, large video screens, and multimillion-dollar construction budgets turn many contemporary strip clubs into high-tech entertainment centers. This is not to say that smaller or "seedier" clubs have disappeared. The clubs in any locale, however, are categorized through their relationships to one another and this system of relationships helps inform both the leisure experiences of the customers and the work experiences of the dancers.

The proliferation and upscaling of strip clubs during the 1980s is situated in late capitalist consumer culture, within a variety of social changes and developments. In many ways it makes sense that strip clubs should multiply during the last several decades, along with the panic about AIDS and fears about the dissolution of "the family." The process of upscaling strip clubs, with a promise of "clean" and respectable interactions, alleviated fears about contamination and disease. The fact that sexual activity is not generally expected or offered in strip clubs also fit well with a growing emphasis on monogamy and marriage for heterosexuals after the sexual experimentation (and ensuing disillusionment for many) of the 1970s. Other social changes may have influenced this rapid increase in strip clubs as well: women's increased presence in the workforce, continuing backlashes against feminism, ongoing marketing efforts to sexualize and masculinize particular forms of consumption (sports, beer, and women, for example), changing patterns of mobility that influence dating practices and intimate relationships, and increased travel for businessmen and more anonymous opportunities to purchase commodified sexualized services, to name just a few.

Despite their prevalence and popularity, strip clubs are still often the subject of intense public scrutiny. Local ordinances have been drafted across the nation to harass, limit, or eradicate strip clubs, often citing "adverse secondary effects"—such as increased crime and decreased property values in neighborhoods that house such venues— as justifications for these legislative actions. Many such ordinances seem to be based on conjectures about just what the men (and women) are up to when they set foot in a strip club. There is endless speculation about drug use, prostitution, and crime—by customers, lawmakers, and people who have never even entered a strip club. Yet my experiences as an anthropologist studying American strip clubs do not confirm the worst of these fears. While these activities surface at times in often scandalous ways—as they do in many industries—I came away from my research with a belief that most of the customers were in search of something completely different through their interactions.

Media and scholarly attention to the customers of strip clubs has been far less pervasive than that focused on the dancers or the clubs themselves. But what is it, exactly, that the customers are seeking in these venues? After all, without enough men willing to open their wallets each night, the industry would cease to exist. As a cultural anthropologist dedicated to participant observation—that is, becoming immersed in the community you study—I selected five strip clubs in one city, sought employment as an entertainer, and interviewed the regular male customers of those clubs. For regulars, visits to strip clubs were a significant sexualized and leisure practice; these were not men who wandered into a club once or twice or visited only for special occasions like bachelor parties. The majority of the regulars were middle age or older with enough disposable income and free time that they could engage in this relatively private and often expensive leisure practice. I also interviewed dancers, club managers and other club employees, advertisers, and men who preferred other forms of adult entertainment.

Most of the regular customers claimed that they knew where to get sex if they wanted it, and that they chose no-contact strip clubs (or clubs that offered table-dancing rather than lap dancing) precisely because they knew that sex would not be part of the experience. While watching the dancers perform on the stages was certainly appealing, many of the regulars were also interested in the conversations that they could have with dancers. Unlike burlesque performers of years past, contemporary exotic dancers "perform," not just onstage, but individually for the customers as they circulate among the crowd selling table dances. Thus, dancers are also selling their personalities, their attentions, and conversation to the customers. Some of the regulars returned repeatedly to see a particular dancer; others enjoyed briefer interactions with a number of dancers. Either way, talk was one of the important services being provided, and conversations would focus on work, family, politics, sports, sexual fantasies, or any number of other topics.

Whether visiting a small neighborhood bar or a large, flashy gentleman's club, the customers repeatedly told me that they visited strip clubs to relax. Part of the allure of strip clubs was their representation as somewhere out of the ordinary, somewhere proscribed and perhaps a bit "dangerous"—yet safe for play and fantasy, where the pressures, expectations, and responsibilities of work and home could be left behind.

In many ways, then, strip clubs were seen as relaxing because they provided a respite from women's demands or expectations in other spheres, as well as the possibility (not always actualized) of avoiding competition with other men for women's attention. Strip clubs also offered the customers opportunities for personal and sexual acceptance from women, a chance to talk about their sexual desires without reproach, even a chance to fantasize that they were attractive enough to gain the interest of a dancer regardless of whether or not they paid her. Some customers wanted an ego boost. As one man said:

> It's just absolutely an ego trip because you go in there, and if you're a warthog, bald, and got a pot belly, some good looking girl's gonna come up and go, "Hey, do you want me to dance for you?" Seducing women is something all men wish they were better at . . . this seems like you're doing it, and it's easy!

Strip clubs were also relaxing because they provided a space where it was safe for those who were married or committed to interact with women in a sexualized setting. The services offered fit well with these particular men's desires to remain sexually monogamous. Customers were not expected to perform sexually or to provide any pleasure to the dancer (beyond paying her for her time), and this was also seen as relaxing by many of the men.

Although some regulars admitted to periodically reading *Playboy* or renting porno-graphic videos, such practices were not as significant or enjoyable to them as their experiences in strip clubs. The customers' reasons for discomfort with other kinds of sexualized services were different—worries about jeopardizing commitments, worries about sexually transmitted diseases, ambivalence about commercialized sexual activ-ities, legal concerns, etc.—and, the point is, this kind of no-contact strip club offered them a "safe" space where this discomfort was eased.

However, because they provided a space in which many everyday expectations were inverted (by featuring public nudity, for example), the clubs were still seen as "taboo," and as dangerous and exciting by the regulars. Many of the interviewees discussed their experiences in the language of "variety," "travel," "fun," "escape," and "adventure" and described themselves as "hunters" or "explorers" despite the fact that their experi-ences in the clubs were highly regulated by local ordinances, club rules, and club employees. Some customers enjoyed that their visits to strip clubs took them to marginal areas of the city. Further, visits to the clubs were often unacceptable to the married regulars' more "conservative" wives or partners.

Significantly, then, strip clubs were dangerous enough to be alluring and a bit less civilized and rowdier than the places these middle-class customers would ordinarily enter. This balance between safety and excitement was very important, for if strip clubs lost their edge or, conversely, became too transgressive, the customers might have lost interest and sought a different form of entertainment.

Understanding the motivations of the men who frequent no-contact strip clubs can help quell some of the fears that tend to drive oppressive regulation. There are indeed problems with strip clubs as they currently exist, often rooted in material inequalities between different classes of laborers, in the poor working conditions found in many clubs, in the stigma that surrounds sex work, and in double standards for men's and women's sexualities, for example. However, eradicating or more tightly regulating strip clubs would do little to combat these problems, which are related to the organization of labor in late capitalism, to systemic inequalities and prejudices, and to the stigmatization and fear that still surrounds issues of sex and sexuality in the United States.

Part 3

Sexual health, wellness, and medical models

What exactly do we mean when we talk about "sexual health"? Is it simply the absence of sexually transmitted diseases or is there more to it than that? Wouldn't a person's psychological and emotional health be a part of their overall sexual health—including their ability to have a positive outlook on sexuality? This might include being un-ashamed about one's body, for instance, or about one's sexual preferences. It might also include being free from harassment and abuse based on one's sexuality, whether we are talking about hate crimes against lesbians and gay men or nonconsensual sex between married couples. These are larger social and cultural questions that come into play when we begin to expand our thinking about what counts as sexual health.

Sexual health can be thought of in positive terms, not simply the absence of sexually transmitted diseases. Instead, sexual health may encompass sexual well-being and a person's quality of life regarding sexual behaviors and attitudes. The World Health Organization, the largest association that deals with health issues on a global scale, uses the following working definition of sexual health:

> Sexual health is a state of physical, emotional, mental and social well-being related to sexuality; it is not merely the absence of disease, dysfunction or infirmity. Sexual health requires a positive and respectful approach to sexuality and sexual relation-ships, as well as the possibility of having pleasurable and safe sexual experiences, free from coercion, discrimination and violence. For sexual health to be attained and maintained, the sexual rights of all persons must be respected, protected and fulfilled.
>
> (World Health Organization, 2002)

Here, sexual health is not just a physical or mental condition. Sexual health is set within a larger social framework and defined in a positive way. It is not just the avoidance of disease but the presence of positive social conditions—respect being a key element in this equation.

Some observers, researchers, and healthcare professionals have suggested that we are on the cusp of a new sexual revolution, one that is driven by public health imperatives. In the last ten years, an incredible amount of research and scientific analysis has centered on sexual health, primarily because of HIV/AIDS and the development of drugs (such as Viagra) to treat sexual dysfunction in men. While sexual health is still largely situated in the context of sexual education and health promotion, the concept of "sexual health" has appeared at the same time that we have seen a major upsurge in dialogues about sexual rights.

For some other observers, sexual health is a misnomer, placing undue emphasis on "health" as a way of controlling people's sexuality. For example, one might ask: Is demanding mandatory HIV testing for sex workers a way of subjugating an already marginalized population? Or, when we think of married couples who might not be having as much sex as they once did—is this just a normal course for a relationship or should they reach for a pill in order to stimulate their sexual lives? We might question whether the concept of sexual health may, at times, function as a way of placing value judgments and restrictions on people. Can the concept of sexual health be both a positive way of thinking about individual, social, cultural, and medical approaches to enhancing people's sexual well-being and attitudes, while at the same time operating to limit our horizons of what is legitimate and "normal"?

Disparities in sexual health

Everyone has heard about AIDS and the need to take preventative measures against contracting STDs. However, many of us think of these preventative measures as a matter of individual choice and responsibility. For example, one makes a rational and calculated decision whether or not to use a condom. Many health campaigns focus attention in that direction, encouraging us to make responsible choices for ourselves. Indeed, this message can be life saving. However, examining how people make individual choices about whether they will live sexually healthy lives is not enough. Many people cannot obtain information and support, and lack options to make the right decisions.

Structural factors, such as limited access to healthcare facilities, or cultural taboos against discussing sex, condoms, or STDs can impact individuals' abilities to make informed, proactive decisions. The more insidious and harder-to-track forces of sexism, racism, and homophobia can also impact a person's capacity to responsibly care for their sexual health. Populations that are not as visible, such as transgender people, may not have as many resources or social support for their sexual decision making. Aging people, who are often incorrectly thought of as nonsexual, may likewise not be able to find, or feel comfortable with, sexual health information and decision making. Therefore, another important way to think about sexual health, according to leading researchers, is to consider sexual health as an individual *and* community condition. In other words, when we are able to think of sexual health as more than simply the responsibility of individuals, and see particular behaviors and choices set within a larger context, then we can understand the more complex dimensions of sexual health as a social question, rather than just individual behaviors abstracted from the world.

A US Surgeon General responds

In 2001 US Surgeon General David Satcher released a landmark publication, *The Surgeon General's Call to Action to Promote Sexual Health and Responsible Sexual Behavior*. The Surgeon General's Report underscored how certain populations in the United States—the economically disadvantaged, racial and ethnic minorities, persons with different sexual identities, disabled persons, and adolescents—face serious obstacles when it comes to sexual health and well-being. These discrepancies, or health disparities, are a major public health challenge in the United States as HIV infection rates, unintended pregnancies and abortion, sexually transmitted infections, sexual dysfunction, and sexual violence continue at alarmingly high rates in comparison to other industrialized countries.

In the Report, the Surgeon General notes that there are disparities in access to good healthcare, in particular among communities of color. The Surgeon General's definition of responsible sexual behavior is not focused solely on individual responsibility, but centers on community responsibility for creating a larger framework of support for people to exercise good decision making. In particular, Dr Satcher outlined the need for:

> access to developmentally and culturally appropriate sexuality education, as well as sexual and reproductive healthcare and counseling; the latitude to make appropriate sexual and reproductive health choices; respect for diversity; and freedom from stigmatization and violence on the basis of gender, race, ethnicity, religion or sexual orientation.

These are very big goals. And perhaps we are on the verge of a new sexual revolution in sexual health. In this Part you will have a chance to explore the multidimensional meanings of sexual health as more than simply the absence of disease, but rather the absence of intimidation; and as more than simply individual choices, but reflective of larger social dynamics.

22 Doctors, patients, and sexuality

Yolanda Wimberly and Sandra E. Moore

Many people think that you can talk to your doctor about anything. But, as doctors who train medical students, we have found some obstacles. First, there are a lot of medical students who are nervous or uncomfortable talking about sex and sexuality with their patients. Second, there are a number of reasons why patients may not feel 100 percent comfortable raising sexual concerns with their physicians. Our hope is to train new doctors to be the kind of physician with whom patients feel comfortable and talk openly. The relationship between doctors and patients can provide a foundation for innovative prevention and education efforts in order to ensure sexual health, education, and rights in African American communities.

In training sessions we send medical students to see new patients with these instructions: speak to them, take a complete history, and do a physical examination. More often than not, when medical students return, they have nothing to report about a patient's sexual history. Students will often say, "I did not know I was supposed to do that" or "How do I start the conversation?" Trainees often believe that a patient's sexual history is something "special" or "private." This is not surprising, given that sexuality is not always openly discussed in the United States, especially in African American communities, where the topic can be even more difficult to discuss. However, sexuality and sexual behavior is an integral part of a patient's complete medical history and it is important that doctors and patients are comfortable talking about it.

A healthcare provider who forms a bond and establishes trust with a patient becomes an obvious source for "intimate" or "personal" information. Access to accurate information about sex and sexuality is vital to maintaining one's overall health. Whether or not healthcare professionals consider themselves experts in this field, many patients believe that they can come to their doctor with these kinds of questions. Healthcare providers' feelings about sexuality influence the way they discuss the topic with patients. A doctor's background and religion may have a significant impact on their morals and values regarding sexuality. If healthcare providers are uncomfortable discussing sexuality themselves, then how can they talk about these things with patients?

What do we mean by "sexuality"?

Sexuality refers to a broad spectrum of elements that make us the people we are. The World Health Organization (WHO) uses a working definition of human sexuality as "sex, gender identities and roles, sexual orientation, eroticism, pleasure, intimacy and reproduction. Sexuality is experienced and expressed in thoughts, fantasies, desires, beliefs, attitudes, values, behaviors, practices, roles and relationships." In the not so distant past, medical schools taught about human life from conception to death but somehow managed to glaze over or ignore the topic of human sexuality altogether. However, over the past three decades medical schools have made significant strides. They have gradually introduced human sexuality into the curriculum—albeit somewhat begrudgingly at times. Whereas some schools now have semester or year-long courses geared specifically toward teaching human sexuality, other schools only offer such information during a "sexuality week." Still, other schools have integrated human sexuality into existing courses. Whatever the venue, there is finally more awareness that human sexuality is an important, if sometimes under appreciated, part of medical school education.

Because educators and healthcare providers realize that understanding one's sexuality is an important part of evaluating a person's physical and mental health, human sexuality education has been added to the curriculum in medical schools nationwide. Sexuality is no longer confined to sexual problems in the specialties of obstetrics, gynecology, urology, or psychiatric therapy. Sexuality is better understood as a part of one's overall healthcare needs.

Medical professionals should be taught how to comfortably discuss sexuality with patients. A general survey of medical professionals found that most do not ask patients about sexuality as a part of the standard medical examination. Oftentimes, it is only discussed if the patient has a complaint related to sexuality. Ignoring sex and sexuality with patients, however, may lead to any number of preventable side effects, including sexually transmitted infections (STIs), unintended pregnancies, low self-esteem, dissatisfaction with intimate relationships, and depression.

Sexuality and African Americans

Despite a barrage of sexualized images in the media, Americans are not receiving information that leads to responsible sexual practices. The United States, for instance, has one of the highest rates of teen pregnancy among industrialized countries and Americans have some of the highest rates of STIs in the world.

Television networks broadcast shows that feature sex and dysfunctional relationships and radio programming is not much better, often featuring songs with explicit sexual lyrics. There is also a multibillion-dollar pharmaceutical industry aimed at enhancing libidos and improving sexual function. Even as we are deluged by sex in American society, it is still considered taboo to openly discuss human sexuality, especially in the African American community.

The relationship between a doctor and her patient might encounter barriers to prevention and education in sexual health and sexuality. There is an unwritten rule in much of African American culture that sex is a private matter, not to be discussed, especially with children. Sex is often treated with the adage, "what you don't know won't hurt you." However, in the case of sex, what you don't know can hurt you—and maybe even kill you. African Americans have an alarmingly high rate of teen pregnancy and STIs. Just imagine what would happen to these rates if there were an open, honest, and, if necessary, religious dialogue around sexuality. Churches are an important source of spiritual and social support for many African Americans, making the church's view on sexuality very important. If churches were to take the lead in educating the community and having an open dialogue about all types of sexuality—there would be a big difference in attitudes about sexuality in African American communities.

If children are raised in homes or church environments where sexuality is ignored or derided, are they truly prepared for the society in which they live? If they are not prepared, then it is the responsibility of healthcare professionals to bridge the gap with accurate information.

Care providers are not immune to social influences. Like everyone, healthcare providers have their own individual ideals, values, and beliefs. Regardless, they need to be able to educate, inform, and advocate for patients. Healthcare professionals must be a source for, at the very least, clinical advice on human sexuality for their patients. This means portraying sex neither positively nor negatively—and always informing patients about the aspects of human sexuality that may impact their lives.

23 Capitalizing on women's health

The myth of "female sexual dysfunction"

Leonore Tiefer

Younger women report pressure to have orgasms every time during sex because it seems to make their partners feel masculine. Does this make their distress about orgasms a dysfunction?

Many middle-aged women often want to be able to say no to sex without their partner feeling personally rejected. Does that make declining interest and saying no a dysfunction?

Many older women want intimacy and physical pleasure without vaginal penetration because it's painful. Does that make their pain a sexual dysfunction?

Do these women all need medical treatment? The pharmaceutical industry would like us to believe the answer is yes.

Through public relations, direct-to-consumer advertising, and marketing disguised as epidemiology, the drug industry is capitalizing on—and exploiting—the public's ignorance and embarrassment about sex, general sexual myths and misunderstandings, and doctors' inadequate knowledge base.

Of course, some women do have sexual problems. And, of course, some of those problems are medically caused. But the fact that most are not is deliberately ignored by an industry that can't yet provide a pill for relationship blues, fears of abandonment or violence, or pressures arising from overwork.

The medicalization of women's sexual problems is occurring largely because pharmaceutical companies and some medical opinion leaders see big profits and big careers in a previously untapped market. If they can brand "female sexual dysfunction" as a clear-cut medical condition, then they can promote FDA-approved prescription products and over-the-counter nostrums and nutraceuticals (such as salves, supplements, or vitamins that don't need to be tested and don't require prescriptions) to the large population of women with sexual complaints or normal age-related, relationship-related, or stress-related reactions.

In the process, though, this could exacerbate women's sexual insecurity, enhance the stigma of "sexual inadequacy," and promote a one-size-fits-all notion of sexual function that poorly serves the public.

What is medicalization?

Medicalization is a social process—both intellectual and institutional—whereby areas of human behavior and aspects of everyday life are brought under the rubric of medicine.

Think of chronic drunkenness. In the past this was a deviant and immoral social behavior. Now it is called alcoholism, a medical condition, needing assessment, management, treatment. Think of shyness and moodiness. In the past these were two ways that people expressed their personalities. Now these ways of relating are called "affective disorder" or "emotional liability" or "social anxiety," needing proper medical diagnosis and treatment. Think of menstruation, pregnancy, or menopause, formerly ordinary aspects of women's lives, now all requiring medical surveillance to check for deviations from alleged universal scientific health norms.

The principal methods of medicalization are the "discovery" and "definition" of new "conditions" that need medical expertise and management. Sociocultural norms (for example, weight, alcohol intake, emotional expression, physical activities, child-rearing, child development, sexual activities) are reframed as health norms, and deviation is asserted to be a matter of concern for health, possibly signaling illness or a "risk" for illness. People learn to observe their own and each others' habits and behaviors, checking for healthy and unhealthy signs. Routine testing is undertaken to search for signs of impending ill health.

Things that might have been perfectly ordinary a few years ago—like women's wide differences in interest for sex or orgasm—are now defined as areas for health monitoring, and biological causes are frequently suspected.

Medicalization has been studied and criticized by a wide range of social scientists who have argued that this process frequently creates misinformation, self-absorption, unhappiness, conformity, and political disempowerment. Medicalization teaches people to think they should all be perfect (and the same) and to look to biology to explain their differences. Feminists have noted that it is primarily women's lives and experiences that have been medicalized, drawing attention away from social and cultural change that would benefit women more than medical management.

Most importantly, social scientists have repeatedly demonstrated that medicalization occurs, not merely because of scientific developments, but because biomedical claims are actively *promoted* by those with professional and economic interests in expanding medical domains.

A prime example of medicalization

Prior to the approval of sildenafil (Viagra) by the FDA in 1998, there wasn't much interest in women's sexual health as an area of medical specialization. There was, however, a great deal of research on women's sexual lives and experiences in the social sciences. Numerous effective psycho-educational clinical interventions, such as masturbation education and body image counseling, addressed women's sexual problems born from the pervasive influence of sexism and the double standard on health and social life.

Internationally, beginning with the 1994 Cairo Conference on Population and Development, substantial attention was paid to women's sexual health by several US and UN conferences, which explicitly defined sexual health and outlined directions for women's full participation.

Research in social science and public policy always cited the deleterious impact of medical problems on sexual life, but medical issues typically took back seat to social and public health causes of women's sexual suffering, such as political and religious oppression, poverty and overwork, lack of education and access to healthcare services, date and marital rape, domestic violence and child sexual abuse, and internalized sexism. The term "sexual health" referred to a broad spectrum of issues.

But in the late 1990s, following the blockbuster success of sildenafil (Viagra), a phase of sexual medicalization entered the media and the health professions like a steamroller. Urologists and others backed by generous pharmaceutical funding suddenly claimed that there wasn't any research on women's sexual health, and that they had arrived to remedy this situation.

These claims were made in the press and at urology congresses, bypassing the well-established sexology organizations, journals, and scientific meetings. These new sexuality experts convened their own meetings beginning in 1998 and established new "consensus guidelines," organizations, journals, websites, departments, and annual conferences in the United States and abroad.

These structures institutionalized a medicalized view of women's sexual satisfaction and dissatisfaction and focused on a very narrow slice of sexual health, "sexual dysfunction." The pharmaceutical industry bankrolled these meetings and structures, eager to create a market among women comparable to that for erectile dysfunction drugs. Ads and exhibits, as well as the content of the meetings and journals, testified to the dominant drug company influence.

More damage than good

Medicalization relies on estimates of high prevalence, and articles about the new "female sexual dysfunction" insist that "43%" of women had been shown to have sexual dysfunction. This astonishing figure emerged in a 1999 *JAMA* (*Journal of the American Medical Association*) paper, which, as *The New York Times* reported, was based on a reanalysis of a 1994 survey, and authored by two people who had served as consultants to a pharmaceutical company.

The "female sexual dysfunction" steamroller of simplistic diagnoses and assessments has now spawned a small army of experts with websites, television and radio shows, boutique clinics, off-label drugs, and scientific congresses, all aiming to profit from women's new opportunities and uncertainties regarding sex. Conflicts of interest are now being attacked by professional and government groups and we can look forward to greater restraint. But medicalization, itself, must also be challenged.

There are some medical causes for women's sexual problems when they're connected to illness, surgery, or use of other medicines. There are treatments already available for such medical causes. However, most sexual problems are not medical. They are the result of sexual fears, lack of sexual information, or factors that, in sexual context, are not sexual at all (for example, anger, fatigue, lack of privacy, fear of rejection). Taking the new sex drugs for these causes is not likely to do much good. Rather, the new diagnoses and new ad campaigns will create more self-criticism and self-consciousness, increasing the market for new drugs but not the quotient of sexual happiness. Worst of all, many women may be harmed by the new drugs as they were by the now questionable Hormone Replacement Therapy.

The only appropriate professional response to female sexual dysfunction at this point should be skepticism, caution, and a renewed commitment to disentangling the science of women's sexual lives and problems from marketing and public relations.

24 Medical abortion and activism in medicine

Angel M. Foster, Jennie Sparandara, and Linda Prine

The advent of medical abortion allows any physician to become an abortion provider. It means that every doctor who professes to believe in "choice" has to ask herself if she is willing to put her beliefs into practice. Physicians are well suited for activist roles, as their profession has evolved to emphasize, not only healing and teaching, but also empowering students and patients. Since the 2000 FDA approval of mifepristone (the medical abortion pill), a new kind of activism based on reproductive rights is growing among physicians and medical students. Through education, outreach, and networking, organizations such as Medical Students for Choice, Physicians for Reproductive Choice and Health, the American Medical Women's Association, and a coalition of like-minded organizations are helping physicians, in all stages of their training, to become abortion providers.

Advocacy organizations

Founded in 1993, Medical Students for Choice (MSFC) is dedicated to ensuring that comprehensive reproductive healthcare, including medical and surgical abortion, becomes a standard part of medical education and residency training. Recognizing that one of the greatest obstacles to safe and accessible abortion is the shortage of trained providers, MSFC works to expand abortion education and training opportunities, foster pro-choice leadership, and develop a growing network of future providers.

MSFC has grown into a significant bi-national grassroots organization, with over 7,000 student and resident members in the United States and Canada. Through organizing lectures, establishing elective courses, and mobilizing for curriculum reform, MSFC activists are changing the opportunities available on their campuses. At the national level MSFC engages in curriculum reform efforts and provides medical students with support, mentors, and supplementary training opportunities. MSFC's Reproductive Health Externship program places nearly 100 students each year in abortion facilities, the annual meeting brings over 300 MSFC activists together to learn more about both the provision of abortion and pro-choice organizing, and the annual Leadership Training Program provides new campus-based leaders with an opportunity to cultivate organizing, recruitment, and communication skills. With groups at over 100 medical schools, MSFC represents a considerable network of emerging leaders in the reproductive rights movement.

In 1992 Physicians for Reproductive Choice and Health (PRCH) was formed to help physicians take a more active stand in providing universal reproductive healthcare for women. PRCH envisions physicians as activists and advocates for their patients, a natural extension of the caregiver role. PRCH staff members have worked tirelessly to promote this agenda to the public, media, physicians, and politicians. Among its missions, PRCH maintains and develops comprehensive sexuality education curricula in public schools, supports fetal tissue donation, supports the training of advance practice clinicians (APC's) in abortion provision, and supports an increase in the accessibility of emergency contraception. PRCH has also joined forces with sister organizations, such as Mergerwatch and the American Medical Women's Association (AMWA), in order to increase awareness of religious hospital mergers and the shortage of trained abortion providers. The PRCH/Mergerwatch alliance has led to the Preserve Project, which seeks to make physicians and consumers aware of the detrimental effects some religiously affiliated hospitals can have on patients' rights to comprehensive reproductive healthcare. From the PRCH/AMWA partnership, the Medical Abortion Education Project (MAEP) was developed.

Training organizations

MAEP was formed with help from the AMWA membership and foundation financial support, and at the request of the National Abortion Federation (NAF) and the Associ-ation of Reproductive Health Professionals (ARHP). It educates physicians, advanced practice clinicians, medical students, and other health professionals about medical abortion. Through varied resources, including didactic slideshows, small group teaching sessions and conference presentations, clinicians can become educated specifically about providing medical abortion. Responding to needs for increased access to abortion and the shortage of trained abortion providers, MAEP helps providers put medical abortion into a historical context and practice. AMWA also works with its student membership and Medical Students for Choice to expand the MAEP initiative to medical students.

NAF and ARHP are two more professional organizations that engage medical providers as activists. NAF is the largest professional association of abortion providers in the United States and Canada. NAF advocates for its physician members in order to help them navigate through the twisted world of medical bureaucracy. The organization also maintains a comprehensive Web site, which includes educational information for patients and providers. ARHP is a longtime advocate of reproductive rights issues, beginning as the physician education arm of the Planned Parenthood Foundation of America. Recently, ARHP has gone public in its efforts to stop current political threats to reproductive rights and science at large with its statement, "Preserving Core Values in Science," a bold effort to forcefully oppose ideological encroachments into science.

Planned Parenthood has long been one of the most recognizable forces in the world of medical activism. Organized around the central issues of abortion and contracep-tion access, sexuality education, and censorship, Planned Parenthood is a catalyst for clinician activism. A new feature to Planned Parenthood's Web site is their detailed vision for the future. Like ARHP, Planned Parenthood articulates the need to meet the challenges of a politically hostile climate head on and has outlined a clear plan for doing so.

In 1998 the Society of Teachers of Family Medicine (STFM), the academic professional organization for family physicians, added a task force or "Group On" Abortion Training and Access. Members of this group have presented workshops at regional and national meetings covering all aspects of abortion care. They host a listserv with a membership of more than 200. The listserv has become an important network of support for practitioners to discuss, not only medical issues involved in providing abortions, but administrative and financial barriers as well. Members of this group have also published articles about abortion care in family medicine. They have made efforts to give presentations within the American Academy of Family Practice, a traditionally more conservative organization. Their proposals have been rejected for every national conference and publication with the exception of the conference that is jointly held with STFM on "Patient Education." To address this censorship, student, resident, and physician members of the AAFP have passed resolutions at local, state, and national meetings asking that the Academy include education about abortion at its meetings, on its Web site, and in its journals.

In 1999 the Access Project, a grant-funded organization, was founded with the mission to integrate abortion into mainstream family medicine and primary care. Believing that a woman's access to abortion would be improved if abortion provision moved beyond specialty clinics, the Access Project has developed a comprehensive and informative Web site. Their Web site includes resources and information for primary care clinicians who need to include abortion services, especially medical abortion services, in the standard medical office practice setting. The Abortion Access Project is a sister organization committed to training more providers and educating the public. Through literature, a comprehensive Web site, and a nationwide network of organizers and advocates, the Abortion Access Project spreads training, as well as the message that clinicians can advocate for abortion access everyday in their practices. The Abortion Access Project also has outreach and activist toolkits, making it easier for everyone to organize around this important issue.

The Internet has become an important organizing tool for activists worldwide. In the field of abortion care, email, websites, and listservs allow for long distance updating, organizing, and training of physicians. The organizations described above facilitate clinician activism by linking physicians with one another and with supportive political organizations. Through their training, physicians are uniquely positioned to take action in the fight to maintain women's access to the spectrum of reproductive health options. Small, dedicated groups of physician activists founded these organizations to ensure that all women are guaranteed safe abortion services. With their help, a new generation of physicians are being trained who welcome the opportunity to provide the full range of women's reproductive health services—including abortion—within the settings of their primary care offices.

25 Bringing medical abortion to rural America

Interview with an abortion provider

Carole Joffe

Susan Golden* is a family practice physician in the rural Midwest. Like most in this specialty, she and her partner practice obstetrics, pediatrics, nursing home visits, treatment of heart disease and hypertension, and so on. Unlike most of their colleagues in family practice, they also provide the women in their community with "medical" abortions using the drug mifepristone (also known as "RU-486" or "the French abortion pill"). If Dr Golden's practice did not offer this service, these patients would have to drive over three and a half hours to the nearest city that has a freestanding abortion clinic, and, there, they would receive a conventional vacuum aspiration or "surgical" abortion.

In many ways Dr Golden could be a "poster woman" for the pro-choice movement and the abortion pill. Since mifepristone was made available in France in 1988, and finally approved in the United States in September 2000, harassment and terrorism against abortion providers has escalated dramatically (Risen and Thomas, 1999). Access to abortion became a major difficulty for many, especially rural women, as the number of facilities providing abortion dropped. Currently only 13 percent of US counties have a known abortion provider (Finer and Henshaw, 2003). Abortion rights activists hoped that mifepristone would address both the issues of violence outside of abortion clinics and the shortage of abortion facilities. Dispensing a pill does not involve the same kind of training associated with surgical abortion; in theory many more doctors would be able to provide medical abortion in their primary care settings. Advocates also presumed that if abortion were incorporated into general practice medicine, it would be much harder to target both abortion providers and patients.

Dr Golden's experiences to date, however, demonstrate that mifepristone provision is more complex than abortion rights proponents had originally imagined. Dr Golden's story is a confirmation of medical abortion's possibility to expand abortion care; at the same time, her story is a reminder that there is no "technological fix" to the enduring social conflicts over abortion in the United States.

I have interviewed Dr Golden a number of times, as part of a research project on the potential of mifepristone to bring "new" providers—those not already trained in surgical abortion—to abortion care. The following material is excerpted from these interviews.

Why did you initially decide to offer medical abortion to your patients?
I had been for many years a strong believer in reproductive rights, long before I became a physician. When I was in college, I was active on this issue. When I opened my practice

*Names changed to protect privacy.

in this town several years ago, I knew that women had to travel for hours to get to the nearest clinic, and that didn't make sense to me.

How did you learn to perform medical abortion?
I regularly go to regional meetings of AMWA (the American Women's Medical Association) and we had a presentation on mifepristone. . . . I realized that I could do this in an office setting. I had met the presenter, Dr Lawrence*, a few times at other AMWA events, and she offered to be my 'mentor'—though she lives elsewhere in the state. She offered to be available to me by phone, to answer any questions I might have. That was really important to me—because there is no one in my local medical community I could talk this over with.

What else did you have to do to get this set up?
I had to buy an ultrasound machine—that cost our practice over $10,000. I had to get new insurance coverage—my malpractice rates were raised several thousand dollars by my carrier, even though these abortions are among the safest procedures I do! I had to hire staff who were going to be comfortable with abortion . . . my partner, Dr. Perillo*, and I carefully interviewed our office people . . . we knew we needed a tough bunch who could handle whatever might happen. We have a wonderful, dedicated staff who are very on board with this. I also had to arrange for backup services from some local obstetrician/gynecologists.[1] That was not a problem—I have lined up several backup ob/gyns. The local medical community here does not want to do abortions themselves, but they are willing to help me in this way.

How has your provision of mifepristone worked, medically?
It's worked great! Very smoothly. No problems at all for the two years we have been doing this. I have never had to call Dr Lawrence about anything. We've been doing about four per week. Only one person had to be resuctioned by one of the local ob/gyns.

How has it worked "socially"? What has been the reaction of this community? Of your patients?
Well, that's been more complicated. Shortly after we started, one of my patients—a very conservative Christian—came into my office, and said, "Dr Golden, do you know they are talking about you on Christian radio?! They are saying you do abortions here, and they are calling you and Dr Perillo Sisters of Satan!" And a little while after that, this prayer group started coming to our office every day—they'd come right at noon, say prayers for about twenty minutes, then leave. They seem harmless enough. But more worrisome, this guy comes every so often, with huge signs, with very graphic pictures— he is creepier. So far though, nothing has happened. We are in touch with the police about the situation.

My patients are for the most part supportive. We have lost a few, maybe six or so, who left the practice because of this, but we have probably gained more. Even the patients who are against abortion are annoyed by the protestors. And my patients seem to trust me. One of my patients—a staunch Catholic—said to me, "If someone is dealing with an unwanted pregnancy, you are exactly the kind of person I would want them to have there, to help them make the right decision."

A divided community

Another incident reinforced for Dr Golden what it means to provide abortions provision in a small town. She was scheduled to participate in a community health fair, speaking about the various choices parents faced with the arrival of newborns. One of the local anti-abortion groups heard that she was scheduled to speak and successfully persuaded the staunchly "pro-life" owner of the building hosting the conference to withdraw his offer. The health fair was abruptly cancelled, as there was not time to find an alternate site. In the uproar that followed, most of the community, including the local newspaper, expressed outrage that the mere presence of this local physician—scheduled to speak on a topic that had nothing to do with abortion—caused the cancellation of the fair. Reflecting on the event, Dr Golden was gratified to see such support, yet understandably troubled by the fact of her abortion provision—only a small fraction of her total medical practice—could play such a consequential role in the cancellation of a long-planned community event.

So what does this brief glimpse of Susan Golden's experiences tell us about the prospects of mifepristone to change the abortion landscape? In some key respects the hopes of the abortion rights movement have been realized. Dr Golden's story makes it clear that medical abortion provision can be safely and smoothly integrated into a family practice setting. And access to abortion for the women in her community—who no longer have to drive three and a half hours to a clinic—has increased enormously. Her story also reveals that another hope pinned to this "abortion pill"—that it would dilute the conflicts over abortion and make providers and patients less subject to harassment—has not yet occurred. For Dr Golden and Dr Perillo, their devotion to their patients and their strong belief in reproductive freedom keep them committed to offering mifepristone. This overrides the negative events that have occurred. But not all physicians can be realistically expected to have such courage. The next step in the medical abortion chronicle, already underway in some institutions, is routine medical abortion provision training in family practice residencies. As such training becomes the norm, and as many more primary care clinicians take on medical abortion provision, hopefully the "targeting" of providers will, ultimately, become fruitless.

Note

1   Such arrangements are required by the FDA, for those providers of mifepristone who do not themselves do vacuum suction abortion, as some 1 to 5 percent of patients will require such services to complete their abortions.

References

Finer, L.B., and S.K. Henshaw. 2003. "Abortion incidence and services in the United States in 2000." *Perspectives on Sexual and Reproductive Health* 35(1): 6–15.
Risen, J., and J. Thomas. 1999. *Wrath of Angels: The American Abortion War*. New York: Basic Books.

26 Aging and HIV

The changing face of AIDS

David M. Latini and David W. Coon

The face of HIV is changing. More older adults are becoming infected and more people who have become infected before their fiftieth birthdays are now aging with HIV/AIDS. These changing faces create new challenges for health educators, medical providers, and clinical researchers.

Even among Americans age fifty years and older, the face of HIV is diverse. In the HIV epidemic has primarily impacted white men who have sex with men. In contrast, older Floridians diagnosed with HIV are primarily African American (47.4 percent), with Latinos (16.1 percent), and women (18 percent) making up sizable proportions of the epidemic.

Older adults are more frequently diagnosed with HIV at a later stage of the disease and they are likely to die sooner than their younger counterparts. Among seniors, AIDS-related symptoms, such as fatigue, weight loss, and diminished appetite, are often misdiagnosed by healthcare professionals as age-related conditions rather than symptoms of HIV/AIDS.

"It is difficult for me to think that HIV is why I feel old or have the problems of aging; and, it is difficult to think entirely otherwise," says Paul Quin, age sixty, who was diagnosed with HIV seventeen years ago. "I feel unable to track symptoms or monitor my health. I no longer understand what might be normal for a man my age and what might come with HIV—what might be a warning."

The picture is further complicated by the fact that there is little research regarding the safety and efficacy of AIDS medications in older adults, including accurate under-standings of dosage and frequency. Medical providers also appear to have a limited understanding of how AIDS medications may interact with medications for other conditions common in older adults, such as diabetes, heart disease, and arthritis. All-too-common stereotypes about the sexuality of older adults persists among profes-sionals and the public at large, making HIV prevention efforts more difficult. The myth that "grandparents aren't interested in sex, and if they are interested in sex, no one is interested in them," continues to be a prevalent assumption in the general public. Debunking this myth is the 1999 survey by AARP (American Association of Retired Persons) reporting that more than 50 percent of forty-five to fifty-nine-year-olds, and more than 25 percent of those sixty to seventy-four years old had sex at least once, if not more times, a week.

Another common misperception is that older adults only have sex within the context of a heterosexual monogamous relationship. According to Florida's Department of Health (SHIP), the ratio of men to women in South Florida is 1 to 7. This gender imbalance may make women more likely to have unprotected sex in order to secure a male partner. SHIP also reports that older males may frequent sex workers, particularly near the time that pension checks arrive.

It is also assumed that older adults do not use or abuse illicit drugs, or if they have used drugs, their use was so long ago that it does not carry any risk of HIV infection. Even the use of prescribed medications may carry HIV risk. Because seniors often live on a fixed income, they may be more likely to reuse and exchange needles for prescribed medications such as insulin.

Healthcare providers may also share these misperceptions and may not assess older patients for sexual and drug use risks, or counsel them about safer-sex practices. "Medical providers often don't ask seniors about their sexual behavior, much less their recreational substance use," said Monica Dea, a board member of the Northern California Association on HIV Over Fifty, a California affiliate of NAHOF, the National Association on HIV Over Fifty.

Seniors may hold their own misperceptions about their risk for HIV. In the early years of the HIV epidemic, research with at-risk groups such as heterosexual adolescents found that many teens who engaged in risky sexual practices did not believe themselves to be at risk because they saw HIV/AIDS as a gay man's disease. Some seniors still view HIV/AIDS as a younger person's disease and do not consider themselves to be at risk, regardless of their sexual behaviors.

"Post menopausal women and their sexual partners won't automatically consider using condoms, since they are past childbearing age," Dea reported. Even among older adults who would like to use condoms, the subject can be difficult to discuss. Because the reason for condom use would clearly be to prevent disease, the implication is that there is a lack of trust in a current partner. Today's cohort of widowed older adults reentering the dating arena grew up during an era when sexual matters were talked about less frequently. They may also have been in committed, long-term marriages where sexually transmitted disease risk was limited. These seniors often lack the communication skills necessary to negotiate safer-sex practices.

According to Dea, sexual behavior for seniors has also changed because of an increase in the use of Viagra. "Viagra is passed around like candy and middle-aged and older adults are continuing to get infected." Viagra has permitted men who have not been recently sexually active to reenter the dating and mating arena, perhaps in an environment of HIV/AIDS risk they do not understand and for which they are not prepared.

The increasing number of seniors diagnosed with HIV presents a challenge to US health educators, researchers, and policy experts to develop successful education and intervention programs targeting middle-aged and older adults. Education campaigns need to increase awareness among medical providers about the risk of HIV due to sexual behavior and drug use among their older patients. Medical and senior service providers alike often require additional skill training and age-appropriate patient or client educational material to more effectively communicate with older adults.

Discussing risk-taking behavior may be difficult for providers to address, even when the older adult raises questions about perceived risks for HIV. "Although it takes only minutes to ask a couple of questions to determine the older individual's risk for HIV, providers often need incentives and education to do so," says Dr. Nathan Linsk, principal investigator of Midwest AIDS Training and Education Center and a founding co-chair of NAHOF. "A number of groups nationally have begun to offer education and information to health providers to help them to ask these questions," and some of these materials are listed on the Web site. Health policy experts also need to encourage pharmaceutical companies to carry out research that includes older adults to ascertain just how seniors react to HIV treatments and how those treatments interact with treatments for other conditions.

HIV/AIDS education campaigns need to incorporate the aging faces of the epidemic so that seniors increase their risk awareness and learn effective HIV prevention strategies. HIV researchers and educators have learned that education programs tailored to the cultural and linguistic needs of particular subgroups are more effective at communicating information and encouraging behavioral change. Lessons learned from earlier research with African Americans, Latinos, gay men, and other at-risk groups provide evidence for the need to tailor HIV prevention interventions to older people in general, as well as develop intervention strategies for older adults from specific socio-economic and cultural groups.

"One in seven new AIDS cases in Chicago are in people over age fifty, and this is typical of urban and suburban areas in the US," says Linsk. However:

> there is a dearth of age specific research and quality educational materials to enhance our understanding about how HIV affects older adults. HIV affects elders in terms of their own possible infection and illness, in terms of prevention and in how they care for others affected by HIV. Good information is needed about how to help them prevent HIV, how to care for their HIV related health issues and how to help them help others.

"I need help monitoring my health and wellness, a way to balance between running to the ER with every shift in my body's balance and letting things go," says Quinn. He continued:

> I also want to help push us all to learn more about what happens as we age with HIV. We can help teach the world more about the disease, treatment options, and possibilities—more about the normal life of the body, its strengths and limits, its weakness and survival. Maybe, just maybe, we can figure out how to control HIV without having it be so expensive, so prohibitively expensive.

Jane P. Fowler, director of a national program called "HIV Wisdom for Older Women", agrees that research and education programs for HIV-positive seniors are noticeably absent. "Older HIV-positive women face a double hardship: the stigma of living with a disease considered disgraceful and the burden of aging in a society that neither values nor respects its seniors."

Overcoming the taboos that older adults may hold about discussing their sexual behavior with their partners and healthcare providers and dismantling ageist assumptions are critical steps in effective HIV/AIDS education for older people. Among the stereotypes about older people, lies a particularly dangerous one: "You can't teach an old dog new tricks." This adage fuels the assumption that older adults are unwilling or unable to change their behavior. However, decades of gerontological research demonstrates that older adults can, and will, change their behavior when provided with appropriate education and interventions that target specific health concerns and provide support for skill development for seniors' real world concerns.

HIV/AIDS education and intervention programs allow providers and researchers alike the unique opportunity to work with older adults and to help them protect themselves against HIV/AIDS, while at the same time extending pleasurable and responsible sexual activity throughout the senior years.

27 No place to call home

Transgender persons, discrimination, and HIV

Rita M. Melendez

The men in the homeless shelter liked Clara*. They assumed she was one of the workers who helped maintain the facility. They never imagined she was homeless. And they were shocked when this young woman explained that city authorities placed her in the men's shelter because they felt it was inappropriate to send her to a women's home.

Clara was born male. The relatives who raised her did not accept that the boy they had known was taking female hormones and living as a woman. For Clara, this was the only way she could live—but it was hard. Unable to reside with her family any longer, she opted to live in a shelter instead.

Like Clara, many transgender women are forced to live in temporary shelters. Besides not having physical homes, transgender people also suffer from lack of a symbolic home in our society. We live in a world where it is acceptable to humiliate and undervalue transgender persons. The stigma attached to being transgender is enormous. Discrimination impedes, not only access to jobs and homes, but also the ability to stay safe from HIV.

High risks

HIV is a concern for transgender women. The San Francisco Department of Public Health conducted a study examining the occurrence of HIV among 392 transgender women (male-to-female) and 123 transgender men (female-to-male). The results, published in the *American Journal of Public Health* in 2001, were surprising and saddening: 35 percent of transgender women were infected with HIV; half of those infected did not know that they had contracted HIV. Transgender men faired better; of those surveyed, 2 percent were infected with HIV.

With the assistance of the administrators and doctors at a community health clinic located in the Bronx, I interviewed twenty transgender women over the course of two months, including Clara. Transgender women include those born male who have had genital reassignment surgery, those who take female hormones but do not get reassignment surgery, and those who dress as women but do not take hormones or get surgeries.

The transgender women I spoke to do not represent the experiences of all transgender male-to-females in New York City or elsewhere; however, their unique stories illustrate some of the ways transgender women are at risk for HIV. In this chapter, I concentrate

*Names changed to protect privacy.

on some of the many ways that discrimination negatively impacts transgender women's ability to stay safe from HIV and to care for themselves if infected with HIV.

What happened to civil rights?

Discrimination makes transgender women especially vulnerable to HIV. Finding work can be difficult and for some, practically impossible. In most parts of the United States, you can legally fire or discriminate against someone because they are transgender. Many transgender women turn to sex work to survive. For example, one person I interviewed for my research mentioned making small amounts of money in sex work that allowed her to buy female hormones not covered by her medical insurance. Many of her clients would pay extra for her to engage in unprotected sex.

Discrimination hinders transgender women from engaging in safer sex in other less obvious ways. The women I spoke to knew they needed to get their partners to wear condoms, but the space between knowledge and action can be complicated. When discrimination is constant throughout life, the need to be with someone who loves you can take on supreme importance, resulting in a decision to "forget" about condoms or to back down when a partner insists on not using a condom. Consider Vanessa* who was recently diagnosed as HIV-positive. Vanessa says:

> We know how hard "the life" is so when you meet a guy it's like you go through all means to keep this man, because you really want to be with him, you know what I'm saying? So it's really hard. You just want to be loved, that's it. Being ridiculed so much, called this called that, being used . . . It's just like after a certain point in your life you just . . . you get needy, I guess.

An intimate relationship may offer a space where transgender women feel loved—something missing from many other parts of their lives. For Vanessa, the relationship ended when she realized that her partner knowingly infected her with HIV.

After the diagnosis

When transgender women are infected with HIV, accessing healthcare can be difficult. Although New York City has a number of services available for LGBT (lesbian, gay, bisexual and transgender) individuals, many transgender women I spoke to did not want to attend those clinics or be associated with "gay" organizations. All my participants identified primarily as women. They knew they were transgender but disclosed this identity only when they felt safe. Identifying with the T in the LGBT was not important to them.

Many women I spoke to discussed how they felt discriminated against by the gay community. One transgender woman said:

> Gays think we are the worst face of homosexuality, we are the shame of homosexuality. . . . But in reality what they think doesn't affect me. I do not live in their world, I don't stop in places they stop. . . . I have seen a lot of discrimination towards "transgenders" and they think many horrible things about us.

The tensions between the gay community and transgender women make it difficult to provide transgender women with HIV care in health clinics that target the LGBT community. Services specifically geared to include transgender people are often not utilized due to perceived or real discrimination.

Taking action

Discrimination in its various forms makes it harder for transgender women to take steps to protect themselves against getting infected with HIV. HIV is a biological reality but its path of infection is social and cultural, one where discrimination lays the groundwork.

Community healthcare clinics have an opportunity to make their services open to transgender women. The clinic where I conducted my interviews was not geared to the LGBT community but was open to *all* members of the community, including transgender women. The clinic had doctors and nurses who were familiar with the healthcare needs of transgender women. Doctors provided hormones as well as other health needs such as HIV medications. The staff was incredibly supportive and kind to all clients and never flinched when learning that one of the clients was a transgender woman—making sure to use the names and pronouns preferred by their clients. Their openness made the clinic a safe place.

Eradicating discrimination against transgender people will eventually curtail HIV infection. We need to ensure that transgender people find homes in our society— making sure that we not accept any form of discrimination in our laws, employment practices, housing opportunities, or healthcare facilities.

Importantly, we need to appreciate the resilience, strength, and grace that transgender people exhibit.

28 High risk sexual behavior among young adults in the US Navy

Genevieve Ames, Andrew Bickford, and Ann Russ

Similar to young adults in college settings, young men and women in the military develop specific cultural beliefs about drinking, using drugs, and "partying." These social environments have been shown to influence the incidence of sexually transmitted diseases and unplanned pregnancies. What remains to be discovered is the degree to which alcohol consumption behaviors are related to high risk sexual practices in this younger age group of first-term enlistees in the military. In order to develop prevention programs that are relevant, successful, and which "speak" to the experiences of young people in the military, it is important to understand the impact that alcohol, along with other factors in cultural environments such as the military, have on sexual behavior.

Beginning in 2002, a research team comprised of cultural anthropologists and epidemiologists at the Prevention Research Center in Berkeley, California began a five-year study of high risk sexual behavior (HRSB) among young adults who were in their first three years of service in the US Navy. Focusing on the US Navy and its unique work and institutional culture, this study is examining important health and social issues surrounding drinking and sexual behavior with young adults during their first enlistment period.

The research team is examining the characteristics of military work culture and the ways in which this influences commonly held beliefs and assumptions about high risk sexual behavior. The research centers on three main objectives, which include evaluating the extent of HRSB among recently enlisted Navy personnel—such as having multiple sexual partners and not using condoms and contraception. The research also analyzes the relationship between beliefs and expectations about HRSB and how the Navy's occupational culture influences these beliefs and expectations. Finally, the project addresses how each of these factors relates to enlistee's social backgrounds.

Most of the interviews are being conducted with young adults in their first period of enlistment. Personnel who serve to mitigate the difficulties faced by new enlistees, such as Navy chaplains, medical personnel, counselors, and educators will also take part in the study.

During their initial enlistment period, many of these young men and women face stresses, constraints, and pressures as they come to terms with life in the US Navy. The Navy presents unique challenges to enlistees, such as deployments, which are comparable only to those faced by the US Marines. Long operational deployments at sea create a host of problems for young recruits, particularly in regard to drinking and HRSB. Enlistees are not only exposed to the rigors of sea duty and life on base, they must also contend with the pressures to "let off steam" during port calls and liberty, and during their everyday lives on land.

It is the intersection of these two elements—duty and desire—which creates tensions that may lead to HRSB in the US Navy. New recruits find themselves in a work environment unlike the civilian world, where strict rules and regulations circumscribe and structure what they are allowed to do—or not do. Navy rules and regulations, including strict fraternization policies and rules of conduct aboard ship, often run counter to recruit's desires and wishes related to dating and sexual relationships.

A key element of this research focuses upon the intersection of strict discipline and sexuality. In what ways do young recruits experience these restraints in relation to their lives as sexual beings? How do young men and women live as sexually active people within the Navy environment? Do constraints and rules intended to curb sexual activity instead promote activities and forms of sexual experience that contribute to HRSB and STDs?

It is important to advance our understandings of sexuality in the Navy, especially given the changing gender composition and the mission of the US Navy. Unplanned pregnancies, which have been found to be highest among women in their first enlistment, can result in costly problems for the women involved and the Navy. For women serving aboard ships, unplanned pregnancies require arranging transfers to a shore job, finding replacements with similar skills, and providing additional training. Many women who have been unable to find or arrange for childcare have been discharged from the Navy.

The high rate of STDs in the Navy are equally troubling. From the Navy's viewpoint, this impacts the lives of enlistees who contract STDs and can also lead to problems in low morale and productivity, diminished readiness, and a need for additional training and replacements. HRSB is most commonly defined or understood as condom non-use. However, this research also examines other factors and variables, such as contraceptive non-use, lack of pre-sex communication (that is, communication about contraceptives, condom use, and status of STDs and/or HIV/AIDS before sex), and the number of partners or sexual history. These factors are critical to the research because they highlight a broad range of issues and activities that may be associated with HRSB.

This study represents a significant advance in alcohol research in the military. The culture of educational and work organizations that involve large populations of young adults (such as colleges, universities, and the military) have not been fully analyzed, particularly in their potential for ritualized and enabling systems for heavy drinking. Clearly, these environments can contribute to undesirable social and health consequences for those involved as well as for families, friends, and communities.

To understand the health risks of the millions of Americans who attend college or serve in the military, it is important that research such as this be conducted. The unique contribution of anthropologists to HRSB research is an understanding of, and appreciation for, the cultural differences regarding which acts and activities count as sex, risky sexual behavior, and STDs. While many public health educators and officials, for example, would advocate condom use as the most significant factor in HRSB prevention, anthropologists recognize that not all cultural groups and societies share this view. To fully understand the ways in which drinking is associated with HRSB among young recruits in the US Navy, it is important to examine all the potential practices that can prevent high risk sexual behavior.

29 Sexual networks of truckers, truckchasers, and disease risks

Yorghos Apostolopoulos, Sevil Sönmez, Jennie Kronenfeld, and Donna Jo Smith

When truckers cross state lines they carry not only their cargo but also their accumulated disease pathogens.

The risk of disease transmission by 3.3 million US truckers and their approximately 300,000 Canadian counterparts is both real and under-investigated. Despite significant research done in developing regions (for example, sub-Saharan Africa, Southeast Asia) that demonstrates links between high risk sexual activity within the trucking sector and disease diffusion, social and health scientists in the United States are only beginning to investigate risky sexual and substance use behaviors of several populations along US interstates.

Dale Stratford and colleagues' groundbreaking study of long-haul truckers in northern Florida in the late 1990s is the first study delving into sexual behavior among US truckers and its links to HIV. Nearly one-third of the interviewed truckers said they had frequent sex with female sex workers and that condom use was rare. A number of truckers indicated that "some truckers" use the services of male sex workers because they are less expensive than their female counterparts and more easily available. Some truckers acknowledged using drugs, primarily methamphetamines, cocaine, and alcohol. Many of the drivers knew little about AIDS, with some believing that it is a disease that only affects gay men or that condoms are of no use. Stratford's study, as well as overwhelming anecdotal evidence on truckers' risk-laden social networks, served as the impetus for our investigation. Here we present preliminary descriptive findings from ethnographies we conducted in Arizona and Oklahoma in 2001, and from ongoing fieldwork in metro Atlanta.

Our research reveals extensive high-risk sexual and drug transactions among several population groups (stationary, transient, or mobile) that coexist in close proximity to truck stops and highways. Informal and in-depth interviews with truckers and their risk contacts in various highway milieux indicate that truckers frequently engage in unprotected oral, vaginal, and anal intercourse with sex workers and other men and women along highway routes, and that they often combine their sexual encounters with drug use. Truckers' use of amphetamines, marijuana, cocaine, and crack—either to stay awake and alert while driving, to get high while partying, or to relax and/or sleep during layovers and rest periods—also emerged as a prevalent pattern.

Truckers' risk networks include a number of varied populations. The nucleus of this network—the male trucker (straight, gay/bisexual, or non-gay identified [NGI])—is often surrounded by female sex workers (for example, "lot lizards," CB-prostitutes, "traveling ladies," US and Mexican brothel workers, hustlers), MSM (men who have sex with men) (for example, "truck chasers," "good buddies," or "buffaloes" [male counterparts of "lot lizards"]), drug dealers, pimps, "polishers" (transient workers who polish the chrome details of trucks), "lumpers" (workers who load/unload cargo), transient and seasonal laborers, homeless individuals, hitchhikers, as well as truck company and truck stop employees.

Members of these networks often play multiple roles, either simultaneously or interchangeably. Every person in the truckers' risk network can offer distinct insights into the ways that these subcultures operate and how this may impact the transmission of disease. However, space limitations do not allow a detailed discussion of them all. Instead, the remainder of this chapter focuses on the truckers (whether non-gay identified, gay, or bisexual) and "truck chasers" (men who pursue sexual encounters with truckers in various highway milieux) because, as a result of their high risk sexual behaviors, they represent the most critical component of these networks in terms of disease transmission.

Despite our study participants' unanimous descriptions of extreme heterosexism in the long-haul trucking industry, our interviews make clear that sexual transactions between truck chasers and NGI and/or gay/bisexual truckers are common. While all of the thirty-eight self-identified heterosexual truckers whom we interviewed vehemently denied any personal experience with truck chasers, the great majority of these heterosexual truckers were highly knowledgeable about the ways that other truckers hook up with "good buddies" (trucker slang for gay men) in "pickle parks" or highway rest areas, brake inspection areas, and truckstops.

For obvious reasons NGI men who have sex with men present a real challenge for researchers. Our knowledge of NGI truckers has thus far been heavily based on interviews with truck chasers and gay/bisexual truckers, located through elaborate websites, associations, newsletters, and events that are created by gay/bisexual truckers and other MSM interested in truckers. An annual convention of truck chasers and gay/bisexual truckers provided our research team with a rich opportunity to conduct interviews and focus groups. Convention participants were almost exclusively white men (mostly gay/bisexual truckers) between their mid-thirties and mid-forties. A number of truckers reported previous marriages and children, while others reported continued periodic sexual encounters with women. Truck chasers reported extensive and mostly anonymous sexual encounters with truckers, some numbering their encounters into the hundreds, a couple even into the thousands.

Of course the idea of men cruising for other men in public spaces is not a new phenomenon and has been documented by numerous sources, beginning with Laud Humphrey's infamous 1970 book, *The Tearoom Trade*. Cruising in the United States has been traced back to the 1890s and was fueled by the proliferation of highway rest stops after World War II. Public or semipublic sex between NGI truckers, gay/bisexual truckers, and truck chasers is a concern only to the degree that these settings can increase the potential for engaging in risky behaviors. While fear of arrest by police and/or fear of homophobic backlash on the part of NGI truckers can enhance the excitement of the encounter, these factors simultaneously raise the level of risk.

Our research suggests that NGI men who have sex with men don't accurately perceive their own risky behaviors, assuming that their straight identity places them in a low risk category. One of the truck chasers whom we interviewed noted that "straight" truckers who were married to women often voiced a preference for other "straight" married men:

> [S]ometimes they will ask you if you are married because sometimes they feel safer having sex with other married men. I don't know why they think they are not

going to contract HIV from having sex with other married men. I think they feel like that they are not having sex with gay men, so it is going to be OK.

This notion that married men would be less risky partners than gay men is based on the erroneous but popular logic that sexual identity, rather than sexual behavior, is the best predictor of risk.

In contrast to their descriptions of NGI truckers, most of the gay and bisexual men interviewed revealed a fairly sophisticated understanding of safer-sex behavior.

Overall, they reported low risk perceptions of HIV-infection from oral sex (their predominant sexual activity) and pro-condom attitudes toward anal sex. Paradoxically, however, a number of the truck chasers and gay/bisexual truckers interviewed also admitted irregular condom use for anal sex, explaining their selective use in a variety of ways: some based it on their insertive, rather than receptive, role during anal sex; others on their sex partner's healthy appearance; and still others on a desire to increase intimacy and/or illustrate their trust in their partners.

It's definitely a trust issue. Using condoms means no trust. I carry condoms, so if someone asks, then yes, I'll use it. But I never take it out myself. I do look their bodies over for karposis sarcoma, drainage, red marks, anything out of the ordinary. I don't do anything unless I can see their body. But I'm trained in health.

This truck chasers' assertion that he can "see" HIV status reveals a shocking level of ignorance regarding HIV transmission. Yet, his admission that condom use implies a lack of trust in his partner raises an equally troubling specter: that some truck chasers might not insist on the use of condoms in risky sexual encounters in order to avoid the implication that the NGI trucker is in fact gay, out of fear of a homophobic backlash. Many of the truck chasers interviewed shared experiences of being physically threatened and/or attacked, sometimes during, sometimes after, a sexual encounter with a NGI trucker.

Our research thus far has only scratched the surface of NGI-MSM trucker/truck chaser networks and issues of sexuality and health risks. At the same time, it dramatically illustrates that as social and health scientists, we need to have a better understanding of the multitude of diverse risk factors that adhere in trucker network milieux in order to create interventions that will adequately educate these diverse and hidden populations.

30 Addiction and the sex offender

Is mental illness an excuse for calculating crimes?

Stanton E. Samenow

Addiction! We hear about it constantly in one form or another. The word is commonly used to characterize a person's consuming passion for a particular substance or activity. A person who loves chocolate and devours a lot of it is called a chocolate addict or "chocaholic." A physical fitness enthusiast who is intent on never missing his daily jog is a running addict or "jogaholic." There's even a term for the incessant reader; she's a "biblio-maniac," addicted to reading. And now there is a book about people who constantly seek to please others, a condition termed "approval addiction."

The word "compulsive" is often used to characterize addictive behavior. The man who gambles away money he cannot afford to part with becomes known as a compulsive gambler, addicted to this pastime. The young woman who steals wherever she goes is considered a compulsive thief or kleptomaniac, addicted to stealing. And so it goes with other types of behavior that are repetitive, persistent, and destructive. They are diagnosed as addictions and considered diseases.

I do not intend to tackle the wide range of these behaviors. My focus is on so-called sexual addiction—in particular the person who gets into legal trouble because of it. The concept of addiction with respect to sexual behavior is really no different from the concept applied to other areas of life. Addiction is regarded as a disease with elements of dependency in which the person with the condition finds it difficult, if not impossible, to break away from the cycle of repeating the behavior at issue, suffering consequences but continuing anyway. In some circles, addiction is conceived of as an involuntary brain disease.

This concept, though, is flawed and is advanced by those who do not understand the mental processes that underlie exploitative sexual behavior.

Take Gary*, for example. Gary appeared to be a successful professional and a responsible husband and father. He had everything going for him until the day he was arrested for attempting to expose his penis to a thirteen-year-old girl. It happened shortly after 3 p.m. when Gary saw the youngster leaving school. He pulled over and parked his car under a tree. As she drew near, he called to her. The girl approached to see what he wanted, thinking he was lost and needed directions. Nearing the door, she looked in and saw him with his pants down. She fled! Not long after the encounter, Gary was arrested for indecent exposure and solicitation of a minor. I interviewed Gary upon referral by his attorney for a psychological evaluation.

As it turned out, there was an entire dimension to Gary's existence that lurked behind the responsible facade. Cheating on his wife, Gary had occasional one-night stands with

*Names have been changed to protect the identity of the individuals profiled.

women, including paid prostitutes. Reluctantly, he admitted involvement in sexual contacts with men. Asked about interest in pornography, Gary first said he occasionally glanced at pictures of scantily clad adult females. Eventually, and with considerable embarrassment, he admitted downloading many types of pornography. In what had become a ritual on weekdays before work, he would leave his slumbering wife and stealthily enter the den, switching on the computer in the darkness of early morning (usually around 4 a.m.), then masturbate while viewing pornography.

Since adolescence Gary had peered into windows hoping to glimpse females engaging in sexual activity. He had exposed himself in the past both to juveniles and adults. With all this going on, he still managed to maintain good standing at his accounting firm and spend time with his wife and little boy.

Gary said that he was "addicted" to sex. It was constantly on his mind. No matter how many sexual outlets he had, he sought more. He regarded the urgency of his sexual drive as a force over which he had no control. But in my professional opinion, Gary had plenty of control and no addiction existed.

Tony*, a man in his 40s, had a top-secret security clearance and was on track to becoming a high-ranking government official. Married and with two children, he was arrested for exposing himself in a community park. Tony confessed to me he had been exposing himself since the age of eleven, but authorities had never before apprehended him. He told me about the careful calculations he made while on business trips. It was easier to remain anonymous in locations where he didn't live and would spend only a short time. He would request a hotel room several stories up but not too high, overlooking a pedestrian area or parking lot so he could be seen. He would part the curtains in his room, but not open them all the way. He would stand naked with an erection in the window but partially hide his face behind the curtain. As soon as he saw someone look up, he'd instantly draw back, and then masturbate in private. He also staked out parks and exposed himself there.

It is understandable that people like Tony and Gary would be considered to have a disorder because they risked everything they valued in a quest for cheap thrills. People would naturally conclude that such individuals are in the grip of a compulsion or addiction—that they must be sick.

During thirty-five years of specializing in the evaluation and treatment of criminal offenders, I have interviewed many men like Gary and Tony. An in-depth psychological analysis of these individuals reveals that, for them, illicit sex is an ego boost, a vehicle for conquest and excitement. Their preoccupation with sex has nothing to do with the lack of a responsible sexual outlet. Like Gary and Tony, most have spouses or partners who are available for them. These men are far more interested in the conquest than they are the sex. One told me, "I find 'em, feel 'em, fuck 'em, and forget 'em." Another asserted, "I don't care if she's deaf, dumb, and blind; all I wanted was her body."

Even with a valued job, a spouse, children, and financial security, these men seek excitement by doing the forbidden. Sex with a consenting partner leaves them restless and dissatisfied. "Take my crime away, and you take my world away," one offender exclaimed. Like Gary and Tony, he meant that life without the excitement of his sexually illicit activities was not worth living. Such a world view does not constitute disease but a preference that results in a series of choices.

There is increasing excitement during every phase of a sex offense—the fantasy, the pursuit, the commission of the act, and the aftermath. Some offenders report experiencing pangs of guilt, but these are fleeting and of little value in deterring future misconduct.

These men know the ruinous consequences to themselves of being discovered, but they have a chilling capacity to banish these considerations from their thoughts while they pursue their objectives. Twinges of conscience are similarly brushed aside.

Sex offenders differ in their modus operandi. Some are deceptive, insinuating themselves into others people's lives in order to extract sexual favors. Once they obtain what they want, they often discard their partners like used Kleenex. Others resort to intimidation or force. Regardless of the method, they share similar thinking patterns as they pursue power and control. The voyeur has a sense of power while secretly intruding into private lives. The flasher has a sense of control as he surprises his victim, attracting or, more often, repelling her. Rape is a raw act of exercising power as the perpetrator reduces a woman to a quivering, pleading speck of humanity who submits and does his ultimate bidding. A rapist recalled, "I brandished my penis like a sword."

I interviewed Gary's wife, Alice*, and Tony's wife, Diane*. Naturally, they were shocked and devastated by their spouses' arrests. Eager to get their husbands help, each spoke to me candidly. Both Alice and Diane thought their spouses were "sick." It is my experience that in trying to make sense of deviant and shocking behavior, professionals and the public use the concept of addiction as an explanation.

Alice informed me that several years ago she had caught Gary with another woman. She left him but reconciled several months later. Chastened by the experience, Gary resolved to be faithful. The couple went ahead and had a child. One day when Alice went to check the email, she was horrified by what she saw on the computer screen— graphic images of women in sexual acts. When confronted by his wife, Gary acknow- ledged he had been curious but avowed he had no further interest in pornography. Alice did her best to convince herself that he meant it.

Alice remained frustrated, as she long had been, by her husband's failure to communicate. But she reassured herself that many men are that way. She also observed that her husband constantly complained about being exhausted. Alice attributed this to Gary being so worried about work that he would go to the office early, even on Saturdays. She hadn't the faintest idea of his early morning forays into computer pornography. Alice's main concern, however, was that when Gary was home, he seemed distracted, like he was in another world.

Diane told me that Tony was a control freak. She was expected to run the household like clockwork, precisely on the schedule he dictated. She was tired of his constant criticism. She could not fathom how he found time to prowl around parks and other public places as busy as he was at work and at home.

Both Gary and Tony disclosed to me how they managed to find the time and opportunity for their sexual adventures. They lived a double life, carefully concealing their behavior from the very people who ostensibly knew them best. The most accurate diagnosis for these men is that they have elements of both narcissistic and antisocial personality disorders.

Like scores of other sex offenders whom I have evaluated, Gary and Tony were making choices. Sex offenders plan what they are going to do. If they think the risk is too great, they resist the temptation of going ahead. The person who exposes himself scouts out the area. If he thinks a getaway will be problematic, he'll wait for a more propitious opportunity or search out a different spot. Sometimes, a perpetrator becomes complacent or careless and takes an unnecessary risk. He miscalculates and is caught. This becomes more likely if he has been drinking or using drugs. Whatever behavior he engages in, it is freely chosen, not a compulsion or addiction.

An offender remarked, "If I didn't have enough excuses for crime, psychiatry gave me more." The concept of addiction as a disease to explain sexual offenses falls into that category. I am *not* suggesting that a person's sexual orientation is freely chosen (i.e. whether an individual is homosexual, heterosexual, or attracted to children). I am saying that people make choices in how they conduct themselves sexually, whatever their orientation. Engaging in behavior that victimizes other people is not a disease. It is freely chosen by men and women who seek excitement at the expense of other people. As one fellow said of his so-called addiction, "I like it too much to quit."

Sex offenders are not suffering from the disease of addiction. They are excitement seekers in pursuit of conquests. They do not have a condition over which they are helpless and lack control. Behavior is a product of thinking. And they think in a particular fashion and make particular choices to do what they do. If the consequences of their behavior become unbearable, they are able to make other choices that are more responsible. Some do, in fact, change their thinking and become disgusted with behavior that they formerly found exciting.

Successful treatment entails a cognitive-behavioral approach. The individual is taught to recognize the thinking processes that gave rise to the irresponsible and destructive behavior. He is encouraged to look in the mirror, so to speak, at the harm he has inflicted in order to generate motivation to change. He is taught corrective concepts. In short, he is taught to become self-critical in a constructive manner. Through the process, he becomes aware of his thoughts, deters the thoughts, thinks of the potential impact of acting on such thoughts, and changes his thinking so he can act in a responsible fashion. With prolonged effort, he can succeed in living a life in which he does not have to look over his shoulder to avoid apprehension. Abandoning criminal patterns of thinking and behavior, he eventually earns the trust of others.

Part 4

Sexual activism and rights

Sexual rights is a very recent addition to the lexicon of human rights. The term "sexual rights" arrived on the world stage in the early 1990s, emerging from earlier discourses on reproductive and women's rights. At the United Nations (UN) Vienna World Conference on Human Rights, the Program of Action called on countries to eliminate gender-based violence, sexual harassment and exploitation [including trafficking in women], systematic rape, sexual slavery, and forced pregnancy. In 1994, at the International Conference on Population and Development in Cairo, Egypt, there was embattled debate over birth control and abortion. However, the Program of Action that was ultimately developed at that meeting described sexuality as a positive aspect of human life, explicitly stating that "sexual health" is integral to reproductive health and fertility control, as well as a requirement for a "satisfying and safe sexual life." While the Program of Action managed to include sexual health needs within the purview of sexual rights, there is no mention of sexual pleasure or freedom for sexual expression or sexual orientation.

Not surprisingly, sexual rights are contested terrain with highly charged ethical questions. In international treaties and declarations, gender and sexual rights have largely centered on the right to reproductive self-determination or freedom from conditions of sexual abuse and discrimination. But other ethical questions pertaining to sexual diversity, including family formations that are not cut from the mold of the heterosexual, nuclear family, are also salient. Sexual rights involve the right to a safe and satisfying sex life, autonomy and "bodily integrity"—the ability to make decisions about one's body, sexuality, and health. Bodily integrity requires access to information about sex, reproduction, and pleasure, as well as a supportive environment in which to exercise one's sexual decisions. Other critical ethical questions surrounding sexual rights include principles of equality, including gender equality, fair and equal treatment for sexual "minorities," and attention to the ways that racial stereotypes negatively impact the right to a supportive environment for all people.

The Internet and the information age have provided new platforms for sexual rights. Vast numbers of people have become organized, visible, and active by linking to each other through the Web. There are forums for debate and sites for people to become politically active around sexual rights, regarding issues such as S/M and intersexuality, for example. There is also a qualitative increase in information about sexual rights. Violations of sexual rights, ranging from rape during armed conflicts or police violence against transgender people, is information that is almost instantly disseminated through the media, email lists, and letter campaigns. While the proliferation of sexual rights organizations and grassroots groups has certainly boomed in the digital age, it is important to recognize the genealogy of "sexual rights" and its intimate connection to the women's and feminist rights movements, and lesbian and gay rights movements from the 1970s to the present. Both of these massive social justice campaigns were indispensable to the development of sexual rights. Activism for HIV/AIDS research and treatment has also invigorated new questions and demands about sexual health and well-being and how these imperatives fit with sexual rights.

While we want to recognize the global dimensions of sexual rights in other countries, we do not want to forget that plenty of questions remain about sexual rights here at home in the United States. Recent research shows that many young women in the United States do not believe they have even the most basic sexual rights. They do not realize that they have the right to say "no" to sex or to tell a partner he or she is being too rough. From this vantage point, sexual rights must also include the right to be assertive, forthright, and heard in these kinds of situations. The right to accept or decline sexual advances and to decide for one's self how one's body is touched is a concern in both the developed and the developing world. Recent research in US schools shows that discrimination, name calling and physical violence continues against students perceived to be lesbian, gay, bisexual, or transgender. An estimated two million students are bullied each year in the United States because they are, or are thought to be, homosexual.

In this Part, be prepared to confront complex questions of ethics, pleasure, gender and racial equality, sexual health, and the right to a safe and satisfying sexual life, remembering that sexual rights are both a global and a local concern.

31 Not separate, still unequal

The Beijing agreement and the feminization of HIV/AIDS

Adrienne Germain and Jennifer Kidwell

The Beijing Conference stands as a milestone for women's human rights. In 1995 the world's governments, with leadership from the United States, adopted the Platform for Action, an outcome document agreeing that women have the right to control matters relating to their sexuality, including their sexual and reproductive health. They also discussed ways to ensure adolescents' right to comprehensive, accurate sexuality education and health services, including access to condoms.

Ten years later, how well has the world implemented the Beijing agreement? And what are the consequences for girls and women when we fail to move forward? While there has been progress in areas like access to contraception, education, and political participation, the most telling indicator is the feminization of HIV/AIDS.

HIV/AIDS rates in general, and for girls and young women in particular, are soaring. Nearly 50 percent of the thirty-eight million people living with HIV/AIDS around the world are female, up from 41 percent in 1997. Females now account for 62 percent of the people from fifteen to twenty-four years old, living with HIV/AIDS world-wide. In sub-Saharan Africa, 75 percent of those living with HIV in this age group are female.

Even in Brazil, where the epidemic has stabilized in the past six years, in 2001 and 2002 the number of cases in girls under twenty was six times higher than the number of cases in boys that age. In Thailand, also considered an HIV/AIDS success story, the epidemic is advancing among women infected by husbands who visit, or have visited, sex workers, with as many as half of new infections every year occurring among cohabiting couples. Here in the United States, women accounted for 27 percent of new AIDS diagnoses in 2003, up from 8 percent in 1985. Low-income women and women of color are disproportionately affected. African American women, for example, accounted for 67 percent of female AIDS cases in the United States in 2003, but only 13 percent of the female population.

There are no band-aids or medical solutions for girls' and women's vulnerability. We are at least ten years away from even one preventive vaccine, and work on microbicides—topical gels or another substance that women can apply in the vaginal area to reduce transmission of HIV and other sexually transmitted diseases—while very promising, is probably at least five years away from a marketable product. A female condom that is less expensive and easier to use than the current model is under development and will ultimately be an important option for at least some women if subsidized and widely disseminated.

But as UNAIDS Executive Director Peter Piot said on World AIDS Day last year:

We will not be able to stop this epidemic unless we put women at the heart of the response to AIDS. . . . The number of women living with HIV is on the rise in every region. Prevention methods such as the ABC approach—*abstinence, be faithful,* and use *condoms*—are good, but not enough to protect women where gender inequality is pervasive. We must be able to ensure that women can choose marriage, to decide when and with whom they have sex, and to successfully negotiate condom use.

Full implementation of the Beijing agreement would dramatically reduce girls' and women's vulnerability and offers long-term solutions. The Platform for Action outlines the interventions needed, outside the health sector, to eliminate discrimination and poverty, sexual coercion and violence, and unequal power in relationships and marriage that put women and girls at risk in the first place. We must invest in programs to ensure that all girls complete at least secondary school and that all women live free of violence, marry by choice, preferably as adults with their full consent, and have access to productive economic opportunities, including full property and inheritance rights.

When governments came together again this March to assess progress on Beijing, more than a hundred countries unanimously reaffirmed their commitment to implementing the agreement. Going forward, national and international financing must be significantly and immediately ramped up to secure women's rights and empowerment. As Noeleen Heyzer, head of UNIFEM, has noted, in 2004 the UNIFEM Trust Fund to Eliminate Violence Against Women received $15 million in project requests but only has $1 million in its budget.

We must also focus on what the health sector can do better to protect women and girls from HIV/AIDS in the countries most affected and those where epidemics are at the take-off stage, such as Nigeria and India. Universal access to comprehensive reproductive health services is the logical starting point. We can best reach these girls and women by strengthening and expanding access to services they already use— namely, comprehensive reproductive health services. Unlike HIV-specific clinics and education programs, which are too often stigmatized, reproductive health services have community support and a head start of several decades.

Donors, national governments, and the United Nations must provide substantially more resources to reproductive health, both to reach more girls and women, and to add HIV/AIDS-prevention capabilities to reproductive health services. If we invest wisely, we will at the same time fundamentally strengthen weak public-health systems. Reproductive health service providers need updated counseling skills and information materials so that they can talk with all patients about, not only HIV/AIDS, but also other STDs, and issues such as combating sexual coercion and violence, and negotiating condom use.

Investments in health and sexuality education must go hand in hand with investments in health services. The only way we can protect today's two billion young people— and enable them to protect themselves—is to shape and implement programs that provide factual information and social support. These programs must also train and educate youth to establish equality within relationships, to end violence and sexual coercion, and to respect the right to consent in sex and marriage.

These investments will build social and political acceptance for long-lasting change. They will also bring an end to the underlying engines of the HIV epidemic—sexual violence, child marriage, skewed power in relationships, and the exclusion of young people and the unmarried from services—which drive unwanted pregnancy, maternal mortality, and wider injustice.

Inexcusably, the United States and the donor community at large, as well as national governments, continue to duck their Beijing commitments and hedge on key HIV/AIDS-prevention strategies, including sexual and reproductive services, protection of sexual and reproductive rights, and comprehensive sexuality education.

In terms of US foreign policy, President Bush's $15 billion Emergency Plan for AIDS Relief (PEPFAR) offers a critical opportunity to reverse this trend and to gain control of the HIV/AIDS pandemic. High priority for implementation should be given to the PEPFAR provisions authored by US Representative Joseph Crowley. The Crowley amendment advances programs to encourage men to be responsible for their sexual behavior; to end sexual violence and coercion, including various practices that force girls and women into dangerous sexual relations (for example, girls' marriages to older men who have had sex with others, or widow inheritance, in which the widow is forced to marry or have sex with her deceased husband's brother); and to increase women's economic opportunity. Equally critical to PEPFAR's success will be the abandonment of the dangerous and ideology-driven requirement that one-third of its prevention funds go to abstinence-only programs.

When HIV/AIDS rates start to fall in every region of the world, we will know that the world's governments have made good on the promises of Beijing. As it did in 1995, the US government should lead the way.

32 The rise of the abstinence-only-until-marriage movement

Martha Kempner

In 1992 the Sexuality Information and Education Council of the United States (SIECUS) began the Community Advocacy Project in an effort to help communities respond to an increase in controversies surrounding sexuality education. The goals of the project were twofold; first, to provide technical assistance to these communities and second, to track controversies around the country in order to gain perspective on trends.

Clearly the most dramatic trend that we have seen is the rise of abstinence-only-until-marriage programs.

When SIECUS began the Community Advocacy Project, the federal government spent very little money each year on these experimental programs. A few homegrown organizations distributed fear- and shame-based curricula, a handful of communities across the country had adopted such programs, and chastity rallies were still the exclusive province of faith-based communities.

Today, the federal government spends over $150 million dollars each year on these programs, abstinence-only-until-marriage organizations represent a multimillion-dollar business worldwide, and students in numerous communities are exposed to fear- and shame-based curricula, abstinence-only assemblies and presentations, and chastity rallies on school grounds.

The need for sexuality education

Programs that receive any of these federal monies must follow a strict eight-point definition that among other things, teaches youth that "sexuality activity outside of the context of marriage is likely to have harmful psychological and physical effects." The definition also describes "abstinence from sexual activity outside marriage as the expected standard for all school age children."

While many adults may wish this were true, it is simply not the case. According to the CDC's (Centers for Disease Control and Prevention) Youth Risk Behavior survey, by senior year, more than 60 percent of high school students report having had sexual intercourse. Even if teens do not engage in sexual intercourse, they may be participating in other sexual behaviors that put them at risk for sexually transmitted disease, including HIV. An analysis of data by the Guttmacher Institute found that among young men aged fifteen to nineteen who had never had vaginal intercourse, 67 percent reported that they had touched a woman's breasts, 22 percent had been stimulated to the point of orgasm by a partner, 18 percent had received oral sex, and 14 percent had given oral sex.

Whether we agree with their behavior or not, we cannot ignore that at some point during their teen years a clear majority of our young people will engage in sexual behaviors. The federal criteria for abstinence-only-until-marriage programs, which prohibit discussion of pregnancy and disease prevention methods other than abstinence, fail to meet the needs of this majority.

Instead, these young people need comprehensive and age-appropriate, school-based sexuality education in every grade. Such programs provide young people with the information and skills they need to make responsible decisions. Studies (www.teen pregnancy.org/resources/data/pdf/emeranswsum.pdf) show that comprehensive education about sexuality—programs that include messages about abstinence as well as pregnancy and disease prevention—can help teens delay sexual activity, reduce the number of partners, and increase contraceptive use.

When surveyed, the majority of adults agree that young people should receive broad-based sexuality education. A 1999 poll by SIECUS and Advocates for Youth (www. siecus.org/siecusreport/volume27/27–6.pdf) found that 93 percent of Americans support sexuality education and believe that young people "should be given information to protect themselves from unplanned pregnancies and STDs."

The funding streams

Nonetheless, the federal government currently has three separate funding streams for abstinence-only-until-marriage programs. The first and oldest funding stream, the Adolescent Family Life Act (AFLA), was established in 1981 to prevent teen pregnancy by promoting chastity and self-discipline. Although AFLA was established before the federal definition of abstinence education was written, currently programs that receive AFLA funds must comply with the eight-points. Since it was established, the federal government has spent over $100 million on chastity programs under AFLA.

In 1996, the second funding stream was established as part of the Temporary Assistance to Needy Families Act, better known as "welfare reform." The federal government attached a provision to this law that established an entitlement program for abstinence-only-until-marriage initiatives. This new program, Section 510(b) of Title V of the Social Security Act (referred to as Title V), funnels $50 million per year to states. Those states that choose to accept Title V funds are required to match every four federal dollars with three state-raised dollars and then disperse the funds for abstinence-only-until-marriage activities in school and community-based organizations.

In 2006 the federal government issued new guidance that required Title V programs to adhere to all eight points of the definition of "abstinence education." By focusing entirely on the less ideological components of the definition which speak to the role of drugs and alcohol in sexual behavior and the importance of self-sufficiency, it was possible for a grantee to use Title V funds for positive youth development programs. The new rules mean that all grantees must espouse the federal government's views on premarital sexual behavior or risk losing the funding. The new guidance also suggested that states focus their Title V programs on young people aged 12–29.

In 2001 the federal government created a third funding stream—the Community-Based Abstinence Education (CBAE) program. The CBAE program is widely thought of as the strictest, in part because grants are made directly from the federal government to state and local organizations.

Many view these stricter standards and the state bypass as an attempt by conservative lawmakers to gain greater control over the programs and messages youth receive. Certain lawmakers have sought to prevent money from supporting media campaigns, youth development, and after-school programs—asserting that such programs dilute the abstinence message.

In 2006 CBAE programs became even stricter and more ideological when the federal government issued a new funding announcement. In it, sexual abstinence before marriage is credited with leading to a happier life, including having a healthier marriage, having more money, having healthier future children, being more "responsible" parents, being honorable and having integrity, attaining a better education, having fewer psychological disorders, avoiding drug, alcohol, and tobacco use, committing fewer crimes and staying out of prison, and having a longer life span. To live up to these proclamations which have no basis in sound evidence and very little grasp on reality, programs are encouraged to rely on fear, shame, and the promotion of biases.

In fiscal year 2006 funding for the CBAE program was $150 million, a 425 percent increase from its original $20 million in 2001. These three specific funding streams, however, do not represent the total amount of money spent on abstinence-only-until-marriage programs. Additional funding for these programs has been allocated through a variety of federal funding vehicles, including special earmarks and traditional HIV/AIDS and STD prevention accounts such as those administered by the CDC.

Why should we be concerned?

Advocates for comprehensive sexuality education have many reasons to be concerned about the federal government's large-scale investment in abstinence-only-until-marriage initiatives. Some federally funded programs rely on messages of fear and shame; deny young people lifesaving knowledge about pregnancy and disease prevention methods; present inaccurate, biased, and exaggerated information as fact; and teach specific religious beliefs.

Abstinence-only-until-marriage programs claim their goal is the prevention of unintended pregnancy and sexually transmitted diseases (STDs) among teens. And yet, they consistently ignore the needs of those young people who are most at risk including gay and lesbian youth, victims of sexual abuse, pregnant and parenting teens, and teens who are already sexually active.

More importantly, however, no evidence exists that abstinence-only-until-marriage programs will help teens avoid or even delay sexual activity. In fact, recent research suggests that some of these programs, virginity pledges in particular, may prove harmful. Teens who take virginity pledges rarely postpone sexual intercourse until marriage and are less likely to use condoms and contraception when they do become sexually active.

Abstinence-only programs in practice

Despite these problems, the federal investment in abstinence-only-until-marriage programs has made this approach very appealing to schools and communities for two simple reasons. First, the federal funding appears, to many, to be a stamp of approval for this type of education. Second, in this time of fiscal crisis, schools are very willing, even eager, to take on fully funded programs.

Abstinence-only-until-marriage programs vary widely; some states and communities sponsor media campaigns, while others fund traditional classroom lectures, one-time assemblies or plays, after-school clubs, and chastity rallies. It is important that parents, educators, policymakers, and advocates pay close attention to the messages these programs impart to students.

The speaking circuit

As early as 1994, SIECUS noted the emergence of a national circuit of abstinence-only-until-marriage speakers, including Pam Stenzel, Molly Kelly, Mike Long, and Marilyn Morris. These speakers address auditoriums full of middle and high school students across the country. During the 1999–2000 school year Pam Stenzel presented "The Price Tag of Sex" to students in Sarasota, Florida; Cary, Illinois; Geneva, Illinois; Butler Township, Ohio; Rochester, Minnesota; Paulsborough, Washington; and other communities nationwide. She told students in Whittier, California:

> I did not come here today to make decisions for you. I don't have time . . . I came here to tell you that if you have sex outside of a monogamous—and by monogamous I don't mean one at a time—relationship you will pay the price.

In Russellville, Arkansas, Marilyn Morris, president of Aim for Success, an abstinence-only program, discussed the "freedom" that comes with sexual abstinence. She and other Aim for Success speakers explained to students "your dog can have sex. It takes a strong person with self-control, self-discipline, and self-respect to say no."

Chastity rallies

Events in which young people pledge to remain abstinent until marriage were originally organized exclusively by faith communities. In recent years, however, schools and other secular organizations have begun to sponsor such rallies.

In 1998, 8,000 students attended a chastity rally in Chicago, Illinois held during the school day and sponsored by Project Reality, an abstinence-only-until-marriage organization. Students carried signs with slogans such as "Save Sex" and "Teen Sex Leads to Death." True Love Waits (TLW), another national organization, run by LifeWay Christian Resources, which is owned and operated by the Southern Baptist Convention, sponsors rallies all over the country and around the world. In 1998 then-Governor George W. Bush attended a TLW rally on the steps of the Texas Capitol and commended the young people in attendance for their leadership. In 2000 more than 600 people attended a weekend TLW rally at Schuyler Central High School in Nebraska. Kate Shindle, Miss America 1997, spoke to the crowd and outlined four steps that young people ("especially girls") need to follow to remain abstinent until Biblical marriage.

Statewide campaigns

Religious messages are not uncommon in abstinence-only-until-marriage programs. The Louisiana's Governor's Program on Abstinence (GPA), for example, funds a theater group called Just Say Whoa. In its skits a character named "Bible Guy" explains, "As Christians, our bodies belong to the Lord and not to us. God wants more for you than a one-night stand. We belong to Him and He has plans for us beyond Saturday night." The successfully brought suit against the GPA, charging that the program used federal funds to promote specific religious messages.

A statewide media campaign in Las Vegas became controversial, not for religious messages, but for messages of fear and shame. One radio ad (www.rgj.com/news/stories/html/2003/08/13/49266.php) feature a girl talking about her boyfriend who wants to have sex. She says condoms won't protect her from all diseases and virgins are less likely to commit suicide than sexually active teens. The speaker then explains that many of her friends lost their boyfriends after having sex and ended up "feeling dirty and cheap."

Opponents have called the shots

Proponents of a strict abstinence-only-until-marriage approach have had a great deal of success. There has been a dramatic rise in the amount of money that both federal and state governments spend on abstinence-only-until-marriage programs; admin- istrations have been committed to funding them; and communities have welcomed abstinence-only speakers, fear-based curricula, and chastity rallies into their school with hardly a second thought.

These successes are not based on luck, nor do they indicate that proponents of this approach have tapped into the will of the general public. When surveyed (http://www. siecus.org/pubs/fact/fact0017.html), the majority of parents, educators, and voters repeatedly say they want a more comprehensive approach to sexuality education.

Opponents have been very successful because they have been calling the shots and framing the debate. From the outset, conservative far-right organizations targeted sexuality education as an arena in which they could successfully affect social change. Whereas they initially called for sexuality education to be removed from school on the grounds that only parents should teach young people about sex, they gradually began to shift strategies. Chastity education was born in the early 1980s and opponents of comprehensive sexuality education saw this as a way to change what young people learn. Instead of arguing for the removal of sexuality education, they began to argue for a new message—young people should abstain until marriage. This was easier for many communities to accept.

The success of the abstinence-only-until-marriage movement is owed in large part to the ability of its proponents to change their tactics and try new messages. Over the years they have responded to many of the criticisms against them. Early versions of fear-based abstinence-only-until-marriage curricula were clearly religious in nature and made outrageous and dangerous suggestions, such as washing one's genitals with Lysol after sexual activity. In today's programs overt religious statements have been replaced with subtle references to spirituality and morality, and blatantly false informa- tion has been replaced with mild exaggerations based on legitimate sources.

Today, the message of abstinence-only advocates is savvy and unified. School boards and lawmakers across the country are presented with the same requests and hear the same arguments: "comprehensive sexuality education encourages promiscuity"; "condoms don't work"; "responsible adults know that teens should be abstinent"; "the only morally acceptable approach is to tell teens to remain abstinent until they marry." These unified messages are reinforced and publicized on the national level by powerful, far-right organizations, such as Concerned Women for America and Focus on the Family.

Turning back the tides

There is some good news, however. In recent years, many communities have rejected abstinence-only-until-marriage education. States have begun to institute regulations assuring that all sexuality education is medically accurate, and advocates on the state and federal level have introduced legislation that supports comprehensive sexuality education.

Students in Lubbock, Texas, for example, have received national attention for their efforts to replace the abstinence-only-until-marriage program in their school with comprehensive sexuality education. These dedicated teens have pointed to the alarmingly high rates of STDs and teen pregnancy among their peers and argued that the current abstinence-only approach is clearly not working. Similarly, a parent in Mt Diablo, California worked to remove Crybabies, an abstinence-only-until-marriage program sponsored by a local crisis pregnancy center, from her son's school. She became involved in this issue after reading disturbing and highly biased information about abortion in her son's notebook and learning that this "sexuality education" program contained no information on contraception or sexual orientation.

Advocates for comprehensive sexuality education have made progress on the state and federal levels as well. A number of states including California, Maine, and New Jersey have rejected Title V funding saying that it is too restrictive and not the best way to educate their young people. Legislators in Illinois, New York, and Minnesota among other states have sought to improve sexuality education by introducing legislation that would require medical accuracy, mandate comprehensive sexuality education, and/or fund such programs. In addition, a number of federal bills working their way through the United States Congress, including the Responsible Education About Life (REAL) Act, the Guarantee of Medical Accuracy Act, and the Prevention First Package have the potential to positively impact what young people learn in sexuality education classrooms.

Moving forward

Unfortunately, by funding unproven abstinence-only-until-marriage programs, the federal government is promoting a conservative ideological agenda at the expense of a sound national public health policy, the health and well-being of our nation's youth, and the will of the American people.

In order to turn back this tide and ensure that more students receive high quality sexuality education, advocates will have to remain vigilant, create unified messages, and take proactive steps to support comprehensive sexuality education in states and communities.

33 Beyond immigrant brothels

The criminal justice system and trafficked persons

Juhu Thukral

At the age of seventeen, Cathy* came to the United States from Thailand, expecting to work off a debt. As soon as she arrived, though, her traffickers demanded the money. If they weren't paid, they said, she would have to go into prostitution.

Cathy was able to escape on her own and eventually found a job in a restaurant, but she was stressed about the money that she owed. Threatened by her traffickers, her family in Thailand had gone into hiding.

When I met with Cathy, I told her she might be eligible for assistance as a victim of trafficking given that she had been held against her will, had experienced threats against her family, and had been threatened with forced prostitution. Unfortunately, in order for adults to access benefits and assistance under the anti-trafficking law, they must be willing to cooperate with law enforcement in the investigation or prosecution of their traffickers. I explained to Cathy that I thought she should explore that option, but she refused. She did not see how going to the authorities would help her pay off her debt and she did not think that trying to get legal work was worth it since she already had a job. She also distrusted law enforcement.

At her job at the restaurant, Cathy was also in an exploitative situation but not in a trafficking or forced-labor environment. She worked close to eighty hours per week and received no overtime pay. When I explained that her employer was violating the law and owed her a great deal of money, she explained that she felt safe at this job and, therefore, did not want to take any action.

Cathy moved through many different categories of undocumented migrant worker. She came into the United States as a person who was smuggled; then, she was a trafficked person because she was held against her will and was threatened with forced prostitution; and finally, she became a worker whose labor is exploited but who is not afraid that her employers will harm her.

Government raids on brothels

Trafficking in persons is clearly a severe human rights violation often involving violence and coercion, which demands a response from the US government. In fact, the Bush administration has in recent years made trafficking in persons their signature human rights issue. Unfortunately, the administration focuses on only one industry: the sex industry. Their official position is that all forms of prostitution and a demand for sex work are the driving forces behind this international problem. The focus on sex work

* Name changed to protect privacy.

also justifies the government's preferred method of addressing trafficking in persons, which is to prosecute traffickers, rather than to examine the economic and immigration policies that are root causes for human trafficking. People migrate to the United States because they cannot make enough money to support themselves and their families in their home countries, and increased border security means that people will take more chances in dangerous situations in order to enter the United States.

While forced prostitution is obviously a severe human rights violation, it is not the only form of labor into which migrants are trafficked. The attention and allocation of resources to the problem are important in fighting coercive situations for migrant workers, but the anti-prostitution agenda behind it is dangerous for a number of reasons. The focus on prosecution intimidates many trafficked persons from coming forward to seek assistance, and the increased interest in raiding brothels where migrant prostitutes work often leads to negative consequences for migrant sex workers and worsens relationships between immigrant communities and the government.

The focus on prostitution to the exclusion of other industries where trafficking exists, such as agriculture, domestic work, and construction, means that law enforcement has prioritized raiding brothels where migrant sex workers are, in the hopes of rescuing them from this work. While this seems to be a good idea, it is actually more complex than it appears and can have negative consequences for the trafficked persons and for migrant sex workers.

There are two ways that trafficked persons can come forward: via a raid, where they are discovered by law enforcement; or by escaping on their own and learning about their rights either from a community-based organization or through outreach and education in an immigrant community. Outreach and education into immigrant communities is a critical piece of any anti-trafficking plan. It is a natural form of information sharing within a community, and encourages people to know their rights and gives them tools to assert these rights. Because the trafficked person engages with law enforcement on his or her own terms in these situations, he or she is also much more likely to want to cooperate with law enforcement. Many sex workers who have escaped from trafficking situations and have cooperated with law enforcement were helped in their escape by other brothel workers who knew that the coercive situation was wrong and wanted to help them leave those conditions.

Raids, on the other hand, often leave migrant sex workers in immigration detention or jail for months while law enforcement determines who is and is not a victim. While the trafficked persons may be happy to be out of the coercive situation, they are often distressed with the experience of having been arrested and kept in detention, and of not being able to work and support their families. Often they are not able to contact their families to let them know where they are. Or they may feel uncomfortable with their families learning that they have been engaging in sex work. These types of raids also create more fear and distrust in immigrant communities, making people less likely to volunteer information or assist people whom they know to be trafficked.

It is critical that as a society, we create safe and confidential places to house people who may have been trafficked, to connect them immediately with attorneys and counselors so that they know what their rights and options are, and to provide them with the opportunity to work and make contact with their families. Furthermore, while of course there are always times when we need criminal justice involvement in trafficking cases, it should not do so at the expense of the welfare of migrant workers. The government's view that sex work is the driving factor behind trafficking in persons justifies such over-reliance on a criminal justice model.

34 Marriage equality

The evolution of a traditional institution

Robert M. Kertzner

"How the world can change. It can change like that. Due to one little word: married." The words of lyricist Fred Ebb in the musical *Cabaret* have an unintended resonance for same-sex marriage today. An issue brewing for more than a decade, marriage equality became a major flashpoint in 2004 and the recent US elections. This one little word, marriage, does indeed raise the specter of major changes—in traditional definitions of marriage, in sexual minority rights, and in the lives of present and future generations of Americans for whom marriage may now be possible.

Although marriage equality as a national issue caught many by surprise, it shouldn't have. Changes in the institution of marriage and in lesbian and gay lives point toward an inevitable union of "same sex" and "marriage" in one phrase.

Trends in marital and lesbian and gay lives

Marriage in Western culture has undergone significant change over the last half of the twentieth century. Increased rates of divorce, larger numbers of cohabiting couples, and more frequent parenting outside of marriage all suggest shifts in the role of marriage in family life. Meanwhile, with longer life expectancies in the West, more adults are finding themselves single, divorced, or widowed. In addition, married adults are living longer in their post-reproductive years, making non-procreative sex an increasingly important chapter of their lives.

All told, marriage, sexuality, and procreation have become increasingly separate in the West.

At the same time, many lesbians and gay men have embraced family life in the forms of long-term relationships and parenthood. To protect and honor commitments to loved ones, lesbian and gay partners and parents have become increasingly interested in marriage as an institution that supports families and the reverence and mutuality of vows.

In Massachusetts the court recognized the importance of including lesbians and gay men in this institution. In November 2003 the Massachusetts Supreme Judicial Court ruled that the state can not deny the protections, benefits, and obligations of marriage to same-sex couples. The court stated that the Massachusetts Constitution "forbids the creation of second-class citizens" and that the Commonwealth of Massachusetts "failed to identify any constitutionally adequate reason for denying civil marriage to same-sex couples."

The issue as social policy

Marriage equality elicits very different views about how the world can—and should—change. And it raises the question: Upon what basis (law, religion, social science, or social justice) should policy be formed?

From the perspective of the social and sexual sciences, research supports the premise of marriage between same-sex couples. Studies have established that many lesbians and gay men create stable, long-term relationships; that predictors of successful relationships do not differ by sexual orientation; that sexual orientation and same-sex relationships do not affect parental fitness; and that children of lesbian and gay parents have the same psychological health as children raised by heterosexual parents. Many of these findings are summarized in a policy statement of the American Psychological Association supporting marriage equality (http://www.apa.org/pi/lgbc/policy/marriage.pdf).

We also know that self-acceptance and integration of sexual identity into other aspects of personal identity are tied to psychological well-being. For many lesbians and gay men, marriage is a joyous affirmation of deeply held aspirations for love and intimacy and a welcomed placement of sexual identity in the larger context of family and public life. These observations, of course, are true for heterosexuals as well.

Studies of marriage also suggest that the public- and state-sanctioned aspects of marriage confer important economic and psychological benefits to spouses and children. Indeed, the whole of marriage is greater than the sum of its parts. Even if you could afford the time and expense to create a master contract that replicates innumerable federal and state benefits, survivorship safeguards, and proxy designations for healthcare and financial decisions, it's not the same as being married, which automatically includes these protections and is recognized across state and national boundaries.

Social conservatives cite several overlapping arguments that emphasize what is *not* known or what is beyond the province of research. These include the fears of potentially negative effects of legalizing marriage between same-sex couples on norms of moral conduct and on children's well-being. Conservatives also argue that abandoning the one man-one woman criterion for marriage opens a Pandora's Box of moral hazards. After same-sex marriage what would come next, they ask. The legalization of polygamist or incestuous unions?

Some religious opponents say that allowing lesbians and gay men to marry provides a disincentive for them to change their orientation, a view based on the belief that homosexuality is a sin or disease. Other more moderate opponents argue that sanctioning marriage between same-sex couples is unnecessary: lesbians and gay men can achieve many legal safeguards inherent in marriage on a contractual basis as permitted by law.

What the future holds

The current legal and political landscape of marriage equality is very much in flux. Recent enactments of state constitutional amendments codify marriage as an exclusively heterosexual institution, while more than twenty lawsuits seeking marriage rights are being argued or appealed in eleven states. Recent legislation and some state constitutional amendments ban domestic partnerships, civil unions, or, as in the case of Virginia, contracts between two individuals of the same sex that suggest the privileges of marriage. On the other hand, recent court decisions in New York City and San Francisco assert that individuals have a right to marry a person of one's choice, that no rationale reason exists for limiting marriage to opposite-sex partners, and that anything short of marriage is a "separate but equal" status that perpetuates discrimination.

Amidst these developments, a majority of Americans favor some form of legal recognition for same-sex couples. According to a *New York Times*/CBS poll, 23 percent of Americans support same-sex marriage and 34 percent some form of civil union.

Of course, that little word marriage continues to make a big difference. Like so many other aspects of human sexuality, marriage is a touchstone for often highly divergent views about what is sacred and secular, personal and communal, pleasurable and purposeful. Some have noted with irony that maritally inclined lesbians and gay men are endorsing more conservative views of sexuality by seeking inclusion in a traditional institution that stipulates the context for love and intimacy.

Perhaps the biggest unknown posed by marriage equality is the potential to discover that married lesbians and gay men share many similarities with married heterosexuals. Regardless of sexual orientation, many adults see in marriage an opportunity to affirm their love and to support their efforts to raise children, participate in the lives of extended families, and contribute to civic and community life.

Like heterosexuals, a large majority of lesbians and gay men want to get married at some point in their lives (as reported by a recent Kaiser Foundation Family study). Many would agree with Evan Wolfson, executive director of Freedom to Marry, who wrote: "Bottom line: there's nothing more human than our relationships with one another and our families."

35 Sexual prejudice

The erasure of bisexuals in academia and the media

Loraine Hutchins

The scapegoating of bi men

Men who call themselves bisexual are liars. At least that's what the *New York Times* science section said in "Straight, Gay or Lying: Bisexuality Revisited" (July 5, 2005).

We often hear this kind of prejudice and misinformation in popular media, even in the gay and lesbian press. But how did a distinguished daily come to such a conclusion? How did the "national newspaper of record" decide that men who are attracted to more than one gender are really inventing their interest in women and repressing a "true" homosexual identity?

The following is an account of what the research underlying this article is really about, and what kind of impact it has had on millions of bisexual people and those who love them. It's a story I know a lot about. I debated reparative therapist Joseph Nicolosi on CNN in 1993. For over twenty years I have worked to educate people about biphobia and how it's interwoven with homophobia, heterosexism, and gynophobia in our society. Still, I was taken by surprise by the *Times* story. *Times* reporter Benedict Carey's article was based on his reading of "Sexual Arousal Patterns of Bisexual Men" by Gerulf Rieger, Meredith L. Chivers, and J. Michael Bailey, which appears in *Psychological Science* (August 2005, 16 [8]), the journal of the American Psychological Society. Bailey, the senior author of the article, was until recently chair of the psychology department at Northwestern University. He lost that position last year but still serves as a professor there. The article questions the veracity of bi men's self-definition, and thus, the very legitimacy of bisexuality as an orientation, at least for men. (Women, the authors say, are not as easily quantified. They've done other research showing *all* women are essentially bisexual, but that's another story.)

What they stuck on the men—a group of about a hundred who were pretty evenly divided into those who self-labeled as homo, hetero and bi—was a penis meter that measures genital blood flow or level of erection (technically called a plethysmograph). No subject was offered film footage representing penile–vaginal intercourse because, as the researchers later explained, they were afraid that kind of footage would be too confusing to evaluate, since they wouldn't be able to tell whether the men's penises were responding to the female or the male or both. Each subject was, therefore, shown several two minute male/male porn films and also several two minute clips of female/female porn. The researchers threw out 35 percent of their sample as "non-responders" (guys of all orientations for whom the lab/wiring/porn thing didn't work to get them aroused). Since out of that remaining group the men who self-identified as bi had penises that, for the most part, didn't get hard during the female/female clip(s), the researchers concluded that the bi men were only masquerading as such and were homosexuals who hadn't faced their gayness yet.

Casting doubt

Further, they opined that since *arousal* in men equals *orientation*, bi men don't exist. The study might have been just another academic paper that never makes it out of obscure sex research journals and sex research conference presentations, but the researchers provided the *Times* with an advance copy of it. Reporter Carey wrote, "a new study casts doubt on whether true bisexuality exists, at least in men." By saying that the study "casts doubt on" the existence of bisexuality, the *Times* moved away from objective reporting and toward taking a position on its validity. (This would not have been an issue had the article simply read, "A new study questions whether true bisexuality exists . . .")

The *Times* effectively endorsed the researchers' opinion, giving the research much more credibility than it would have otherwise had. The story made its way into other news media outlets and was reprinted and commented on around the world. The researchers also were strategic, or perhaps just lucky, to get the story into the *Times* the same week a major sex research conference was occurring in Ottawa, The International Academy of Sex Research (IASR), thus assuring even more publicity for their assertions.

When the Gay and Lesbian Alliance Against Defamation (GLAAD) challenged the *Times* about its inflammatory headline, their response was that "straight, gay or lying" is a well known idiomatic comment gays make about bisexuals, and therefore was appropriate. Thinking this line of reasoning could sanction a lot more inaccuracies and hate speech, GLAAD requested that the *Times* at least change this article's headline on their Web site. They refused to do so. GLAAD issued a statement and mounted an online campaign to help mobilize people's response.

The organized response

Within twenty-four hours of the article's release an ad hoc coalition of LGBT activists and academics came together, under the leadership of the National Gay and Lesbian Task Force, to coordinate a national response. The Task Force prepared, and posted on its Web site, critiquing the study the article was based upon. More importantly, they enlisted BiNet USA: The National Bisexual Network, the Bisexual Resource Center of Boston, and GLAAD in a series of nationwide conference calls that helped strategize a way to hold the *Times* accountable for its hate speech and misinformation. At least one group beyond the LGBT community—the progressive media watchdog group Fairness and Accuracy In Reporting (FAIR)—also issued a statement protesting the *Times'* handling of the research.

A week later, amidst a flurry of criticism, the *Times* published a small selection of the many letters they had received on the article. The only published letter defending the article was by conservative gay writer Chandler Burr, who contributes to the *Times*.

The story continued to grow legs well into the second and third weeks after its initial release. While it remained one of the *Times'* Web site most forwarded articles for more than two weeks, the *Philadelphia Inquirer* and *Los Angeles Times* covered public response to the story and asked additional questions about the research's original content. Increasing media response came from blogs of all sorts, bisexual listservs, websites, LGBT magazines, and local newspapers around the English-speaking world— with reprints and discussions from Belfast to Baltimore, Toronto to Atlanta, Sydney to Seattle, and many points in between. Meanwhile, the ad hoc coalition moved ahead with plans to arrange a meeting with the editor of the *New York Times* science section to discuss the coverage of the research and their future coverage of bisexuality and other sexual orientation/identity issues. A meeting did finally take place on July 27, 2005. There, coalition representatives aired their concerns and suggestions, and the *Times* promised to take these into consideration in future reporting.

The research flaws

The Task Force, with input from LGBT academics who had read advance copies of the Bailey *et al.* study, developed a preliminary fact sheet. It points out that the *Times* fails "to note several serious and obvious questions about the study's methodology and underlying premises" and also "misstates some of the study's conclusions." As the Task Force writers said, the assertion by Bailey, Rieger, and Chivers that arousal, at least in men, equals sexual orientation, is a ridiculous oversimplification of the complexity of sexual desire. Rather, arousal is "a combination of cognitive and physical responses, not reducible to genital responses to pornography."

They also questioned the validity of the plethysmograph. The controversial device was developed in Eastern Europe during the 1950s and brought to Canada and the United States soon thereafter. It has been used to measure sexual response in relation to screening-out alleged homosexuals from those seeking government service or citizenship. The Task Force fact sheet further asked how seriously one could take any study that had to throw out 35 percent of its respondents as non-responders (those men who had no measurable erections while watching the films), and pointed out that the researchers said that this study was part of a larger group of other such studies but that it really was not.

In addition to the above methodological problems, the fact sheet noted "many serious controversies that have plagued one of the study's authors" (Bailey). The *New York Times* didn't mention that Bailey's research reputation has been seriously questioned. As the Task Force efforts continued, it became increasingly clear that the controversy over his past writings and research methods was wide indeed.

Bailey made an unwelcome name for himself within the transgender community several years ago, culminating in the 2003 publication of his book about trans women, *The Man Who Would Be Queen*. When *The Man Who Would Be Queen* came out *Publishers Weekly* said that:

> Bailey's scope is so broad that when he gets down to pivotal constructs, as in detailing the data of scientific studies such as Richard Green's about "feminine boys" or Dean Hamer's work on the so-called "gay gene," the material is vague, and not cohesive. Bailey tends towards overreaching, unsupported generalizations, such as his claim that "regardless of marital laws there will always be fewer gay men who are romantically attached" or that the African-American community is "a relatively anti-gay ethnic minority." Add to this the debatable supposition that innate "masculine" and "feminine" traits, in the most general sense of the words, decidedly exist, and his account as a whole loses force.

Since the book came out Northwestern University received many complaints from transsexual women Bailey interviewed, who complained that they didn't know he was using them as research subjects, and that distorted versions of their case histories would appear in his book. Northwestern opened a formal investigation into charges of research misconduct against Bailey, as reported in a series of articles in the *Daily Northwestern* and the *Chronicle of Higher Education*. In October 2004 Bailey resigned from his chairmanship of the psychology department, following the completion of the investigation and implementation of undisclosed sanctions against him by the university (*Chronicle of Higher Education*, December 10, 2004).

Sexuality research: the larger picture

The Bailey, Rieger, Chiver research is part of a long line of studies that look for a genetic link to sexual orientation, as developed most recently by Dean Hamer, Simon LeVay, *et al.* In an interesting yet probably totally unintended coincidence, the national gay news magazine *The Advocate* came out with a related cover story on July 5, 2005 the same day the *New York Times* released "Straight, Gay or Lying." *The Advocate*'s story, "Scents and Sexuality," by Lisa Neff, reports on new studies about sexual orientation and smell. She then segues into a summary of genetics and sexual orientation studies over the past hundred years. While the survey article is quite well done, it overlooks bisexual, transgender, and intersex people and the increasing body of research developed on them in the past twenty years. Why does this disconnect still exist? There's no simple answer. However, examining the origins of sexual orientation research does provide some clues.

Psychologists look at sexual orientation in two essentially different ways: the dichotomous approach (that which is not heterosexual is homosexual) and the more multidimensional approach, which views orientation more as a spectrum than two separate and distinct poles. Of course, the best known example of this spectrum view is the Kinsey scale, which encompasses a range from exclusively heterosexual (0) to exclusively homosexual (6), with most people falling somewhere in between.

According to bisexual psychologist and author Ron Fox, the field has been evolving through a three stage reinterpretation of sexual orientation since the early 1970s when therapists stopped seeing homosexuality as an illness. At the first stage it's fine to be lesbian or gay since homosexuality is no longer an illness, but sexual orientation itself is still seen as dichotomous, either/or, same sex *or* different sex oriented, with nothing in between. Most of psychology has now moved beyond that stage and sees dichotomous sexual orientation as too simplistic. At this second stage bisexuality is recognized as a legitimate orientation. This stage also reflects the point at which gay organizations began adding bisexual to their names, as in LGB. When the multidimensionality of sexual orientation is sufficiently explored it becomes clear that gender identity and expression, as well, exist along a similar continuum rather than only at two poles. This is the third stage, where, as a result of lesbian, gay, bisexual, and transgender psychologists working together with heterosexuals to develop a more complex understanding of sexual orientation, the same complex understanding of gender becomes integrated into how psychology and sexuality research is conducted and taught.

And this new, more nuanced understanding of both sexual orientation and gender as spectrums isn't only confined to the research field. Activists and educators must often position their media advocacy and public sexuality education work in the gap between the old dichotomous view of sexual orientation and the newer, more multidimensional one. As they do this they hone classic bisexual skills, particularly the roles of bridge builder and diplomat. It is their talent to move back and forth—translating between groups and different sets of ideas, interpreting each to the other, and helping everyone see we're not so far apart as it seems—that helps them survive with their identities and integrity intact. A positive outcome from the *New York Times* article is the coordinated effort to critique Bailey *et al.*'s research.

This particular story of how we responded to one article elapsed over a mere month in time. But the larger picture of how this experience relates to other queer stories with unexplored bi angles remains to be told. We look forward to discussions on related topics such as: the developing definition of bisexual orientation, the relationship between transgender and bisexual identities, and ex-gay reparative/conversion therapy and its connection to bisexuality. All of this and more came up in our brainstorming around how to respond to the *New York Times*. It's been a valuable learning experience, one that has provided some sense of comfort and accomplishment to counterbalance the underlying pain and human suffering for bisexuals and those who love us that the publication of the *Times*' "Straight, Gay or Lying" story initially exposed.

36 Seeking help in rural communities

Homophobia and racism impact mental healthcare

Cathleen Willging, Lisa Cacari-Stone,
Louise Lamphere, Rae Lewis, and Bonnie Duran

Karen*, an Anglo woman from the urban West Coast, moved to a rural community in New Mexico four years ago. Her partner, Mary*, an American Indian woman, was from the area and had family there. Karen was an underpaid school teacher, while Mary worked odd jobs. Terrified about losing her teaching position—the couple's main source of income—Karen let few people know that she was a lesbian. The transition from urban to rural life was not easy for Karen, who became despondent and socially isolated. While Mary did her best to help Karen adjust to the new surroundings, Karen remained emotionally distressed and, occasionally, was suicidal.

Two years ago Karen decided to get professional help, settling on a mental health provider available at no cost through the Employee Assistance Program at work. Karen felt "violated" by this encounter, however. During her one and only session, the provider unashamedly revealed that his clinical knowledge of homosexuality derived from an abnormal psychology class that he took more than thirty years ago. He then went on to disparage Karen for being a lesbian and to insinuate that her partner, Mary, must be an alcoholic since she was American Indian. Furthermore, because Karen opted to be in an interracial relationship with a woman and to live in a rural area, the provider opined that it was simply "too much" to ask other people in the community "to swallow" her "lifestyle choice." Though she still felt depressed, Karen refused to see other local providers in the years that followed.

Karen's story is not unique. We conducted in-depth interviews with thirty-eight lesbian, gay, bisexual, and transgender (LGBT) people in rural New Mexico about how they tried to access professional services for their mental health problems. These discussions were supplemented with in-depth interviews with twenty mental health providers who both live and practice in rural communities. From these discussions, we learned that fear, loneliness, and off-putting interactions within heteronormative treatment settings were common themes in the help-seeking experiences of LGBT people in rural areas. The cultural ideal of "self-reliance" (preference to solve emotional problems on one's own) and the view of mental illness as a "weakness" or personal shortcoming were often strong in rural communities, discouraging LGBT people from

*Names changed to protect privacy.

getting care. Leroy*, an American Indian gay man and lifelong rural resident, was overcome with grief after losing his aunt, but it took him more than one year to break free from this stigma and make an appointment with a mental health provider. The provider, however, "laughed" in disbelief when Leroy said that he was gay, causing them both discomfort during their session together.

Money, distance, and stigma make it hard for rural LGBT people, like Karen and Leroy, to get LGBT-affirmative services. Social support networks, composed of family and friends, and informal mental health resources, including those found in indigenous healing systems, often serve as alternatives to professional mental healthcare. In lieu of counseling, for example, Karen and Mary turned to American Indian traditional healers, who offered prayers and advice that aided them in their everyday dealings with people in the broader community. Mary's own parents and members of her extended family also provided unwavering support to both women. Similarly, at the urging of his extended family, Leroy consulted with a traditional healer, whom he credited with helping him grapple with his grief and depression, while affirming his personhood.

Our limited knowledge about LGBT mental health

The combination of prejudice and discrimination hampers both research and services targeting the mental health of LGBT people. The federal government's historical disinterest in supporting studies concerning LGBT issues and more recent political pressure have limited research regarding these traditionally underserved groups. Some researchers also worry about being marginalized in scholarly communities if they center their work on LGBT people. Additionally, the methodological challenges of undertaking such research are quite considerable. These challenges include lack of personal identification among potential participants with externally imposed social categories, such as "lesbian," "gay," "bisexual," and "transgender," and the problem of recruiting "hidden" populations to take part in studies on sensitive topics. These challenges increase substantially in rural areas, where individual privacy and confidentiality are highly valued and people are more likely to conceal their LGBT identities and mental health problems in order to sidestep community gossip.

As a result of such challenges, we know little about the mental health needs of LGBT people. However, findings published in 2001 from the National Comorbidity Survey— one of the largest population-based epidemiological studies of mental illness undertaken in the United States—clearly show that LGBT people are at increased risk for psychiatric problems.

Anti-LGBT discrimination and violence can trigger mental distress and illness, alcohol and drug abuse, and even suicide. Discrimination may affect the employment, housing, and healthcare opportunities of LGBT people, making them especially susceptible to adverse mental health outcomes. "Hate crimes," which encompass threats and acts of violence against LGBT people, occur in schools, homes, work, and public spaces, and are carried out by family members as well as strangers. In the rural area where Karen and Leroy live, "hate crimes" remain underreported or are simply ignored by the legal authorities. The effect of discrimination and violence may be exacerbated in rural areas, where mental healthcare and basic social services are often insufficient for the general population and virtually nonexistent for LGBT people.

What we do know about LGBT mental health issues is based mostly on research involving convenience samples of self-identified gay men and lesbians who are white, middle class, educated, and urban or suburban—rather than racial and ethnic minorities, poor or working-class individuals, and people who reside in rural settings. Of 124 lesbian, gay, and bisexual specific articles published in American Psychological Association journals over a ten-year period, only six pertained to people of color (Harper, Jernewall, and Zea, 2004). The way we talk about "coming out" processes or LGBT identity formation has been shaped by studies that privilege the experiences of the dominant group. The available research underscores that discrimination associated with sexual orientation and gender non-conformity can have a damaging effect on a person's mental health. This research, however, does not accurately reflect the experiences of people of color for whom multiple layers of oppression based on race, ethnicity, and socioeconomic status, in addition to gender and sexuality may take a greater toll. The complicated ways in which these intersecting issues affect the mental health of rural people of color is a topic that is woefully understudied.

Access problems and quality of care

Although lack of healthcare coverage pervades LGBT populations in this country, this problem is even greater in rural areas, where local economies are in sharp decline and rates of unemployment and uninsurance are escalating. The largely rural state of New Mexico has one of the highest rates of poverty in the nation. Poverty increases one's risk for developing a mental health problem, while uninsurance makes it all that much harder to get care. The costs of care are a likely deterrent for rural LGBT people in need of professional mental health services.

As suggested in the Healthy People 2010 Companion Document for LGBT Health, a supplement to the federal government's blueprint for public health published by the Gay and Lesbian Medical Association in 2001, rural LGBT people may experience specific and unique stress related to disclosure. They may be afraid of having their sexual orientation or gender identity revealed along with their mental health status. They may also fear losing their job, as was Karen's concern, or their house or apartment. Furthermore, rural LGBT people may internalize homophobic (as well as racist) beliefs and attitudes espoused by other people in their communities; this can also contribute to self-devaluation.

Because of these substantial access barriers and everyday stressors, the decision to seek out mental healthcare does not always come easily for rural LGBT people. For example, Serena*, a transgender Hispanic woman, refused to get services from her community's local mental health clinic because the providers there "look at you or make you feel like you're dirty."

LGBT clients may encounter negative reactions from mental health providers, from overt forms of hostility and intolerance to subtle forms of bias. Underlying these reactions is the historical role that the mental health professions have played in reinforcing negative societal attitudes and beliefs about LGBT people. The psychiatric profession played a dominant role in promoting the view of "homosexuality" as a mental disease. The label sanctioned societal discrimination against LGBT people. The American Psychiatric Association (APA) officially expunged "homosexuality" from its list of diagnosable illnesses in the 1970s and in subsequent decades issued professional practice codes that prohibit LGBT discrimination. (The diagnosis of Gender Identity Disorder was not removed, however.) The APA even asserted that the alignment of providers with lingering anti-LGBT societal attitudes and behaviors can reinforce self-hatred already experienced by lesbian, gay, and bisexual clients, and cause harm to them during treatment. Other professional associations, including the American Psychological Association and the National Association of Social Workers, followed suit with the adoption of similar position statements and practice codes. Without enforcement, however, these codes are ineffectual in countering negative therapeutic practices, including the practice of now debunked "reparative" or "conversion" therapies to assimilate clients into heteronormative lifestyles.

Lack of accurate, contemporary knowledge about LGBT people and heterosexist bias may lead some rural mental health providers to base their decisions about clinical assessment and treatment based on outmoded models. One such model is the "deficits paradigm," in which "sick" people (LGBT individuals) must assimilate into "normality" (a heterosexual lifestyle) to achieve mental wellness. Most tellingly, Eric*, an Anglo provider at a rural residential treatment center, explained how his colleagues would sometimes let clients know that they did not think it was okay for them to be LGBT: "If they would get over that, things would fall into place."

Rural mental health and substance-abuse treatment facilities commonly lack LGBT providers, despite growing evidence suggesting that LGBT clients are more apt to take part in programs that address LGBT issues and less likely to comply with treatment from homophobic providers. On the flip side, however, some rural providers are fearful of gossip and disapproving judgment if their own LGBT status becomes publicly known, an admission that can result in decreased client referrals and caseloads.

LGBT clients who do make use of available services may risk rejection from fellow clients, particularly when they take part in treatment that relies on group therapies. Elena*, an American Indian provider, reported that clients went "haywire" when a woman mentioned that she was a lesbian during group therapy. Providers may also discourage LGBT clients from broaching their sexuality and gender issues and do not necessarily quell the negative reactions of non-LGBT clients when such issues are raised. Their failure to address these reactions enables hostile attitudes to thrive, while ultimately diminishing the effectiveness of group therapy.

It takes a community

Without access to LGBT-supportive mental healthcare and support organizations, some rural LGBT individuals may experience heightened feelings of social isolation and mental distress. Such is the case for Karen, who lost her LGBT friends and contacts when she moved to a rural area. For those who grow up in such areas, lack of LGBT-specific information and ties to other LGBT people can also hinder the development of an affirmative sense of self.

Yet, unique protective mechanisms operate among LGBT populations in rural settings. For example, social bonds and supportive relationships are considered to be essential to the maintenance of positive mental health. In the LGBT population at large, researchers have found that strong family connections, including a close relationship with a parent or accepting relative, attachment to external support systems (for example, church, school, community group), and well developed social networks can all help prevent LGBT people from developing mental health problems. Likewise, these connections can contribute to recovery. For example, in an effort to overcome his addiction to methamphetamine, Lorenzo*, a Hispanic gay man, swore off his anonymity, moving from a metropolitan area with a large LGBT population to receive emotional support from his family within the rural community where he was born and raised.

Cultural factors influence experiences of mental distress and help-seeking among rural LGBT populations. As noted previously, such factors shape ideas about "self-reliance" and concerns about confidentiality that can inhibit rural residents from accessing professional services. However, LGBT people can draw upon a broad range of mental health resources that are available in rural communities, but which are not typically associated with professional treatment systems and, moreover, are oftentimes devalued or misunderstood by providers working within these systems. The use of *curanderismo* and other cultural healing practices, for instance, is pervasive among rural Hispanics in New Mexico. Traditional medicine and alternative therapies are widely used among rural American Indians, including self-identified LGBT people—some of whom assume culturally sanctioned roles as health practitioners within the healing systems of their societies.

Religiosity and spiritually based healing practices among African American, Hispanic, and American Indian populations are associated with enhanced health status, and may play a constructive role promoting positive mental health for LGBT people living in otherwise medically underserved rural environments. Understanding the importance of such protective mechanisms is necessary terrain to be covered in future LGBT mental health services research.

In order to understand the social dynamics of how at-risk groups of rural LGBT people creatively and effectively address mental health problems, we must acknowledge the critical functions of social support networks, nonprofessional healing systems, and informal resources. At the same time, we must take stock of the experiences of those rural LGBT people who do seek services within professional treatment systems. Even though we did learn of clinical settings where services were rendered responsibly and misconceptions about LGBT mental health issues were not condoned, the experiences of rural residents, such as Karen and Leroy, attest to the fact that immediate steps must be taken to ensure that all LGBT people can benefit from quality care.

Reference

Harper, G.W., N. Jernewall, and M.C. Zea. 2004. "Giving voice to emerging science and theory for lesbian, gay, bisexual people of color." *Cultural Diversity and Ethnic Minority Psychology* 10(3): 187–199.

Acknowledgment: This article was funded by grants from the National Institute of Mental Health (1R21 MH068628–01 and 1R03 MH65564). We thank Nancy Nelson for her helpful comments on an earlier draft.

37 Disability and sexuality

From medical model to sexual rights

Russell P. Shuttleworth

Everyone agrees sexuality is an important part of life. But when I told people that my doctoral research focused on the sexual narratives of men with cerebral palsy, it was not uncommon for non-disabled people to ask, "Can they do that?" The people who asked this question were not unintelligent, but they had bought into the myth that disabled people are asexual. Unfortunately, the Disability Rights Movement and academic disability studies have been slow to politicize disability and sexuality. As Barbara Waxman, a disabled feminist activist and scholar, charged in the pages of the *Disability Rag* in 1991:

> the disability rights movement has never addressed sexuality as a key political issue, though many of us find sexuality to be the area of our greatest oppression. We are more concerned with being loved and finding sexual fulfillment than in getting on the bus.

There are a wide range of issues related to disability and sexuality that deserve social and political attention, including sexual abuse, asexual and hypersexual media images of disabled people, disability and gender issues, sexual identity and orientation, interpersonal barriers and sexual intimacy, the use of sex workers and sexual surrogates, facilitated sex, and barriers to sexual access for significantly disabled persons living in institutions and group homes. Although activists and researchers have begun to politicize these issues, disabled people continue to confront ignorance about their sexual potential and face sexual oppression in their everyday lives. By considering the history of the disability community's politicization of these issues, we are able to develop research and advocacy strategies that will effectively dispel the myth of disabled people as asexual.

The disability and sexuality research of the 1950s through much of the 1970s was generated in response to the loss of sexual function and/or sensation by heterosexual men who were disabled in early to mid-adulthood because of a major physical trauma, often a spinal cord injury. These men were sexually compromised in varying degrees depending on the location of the injury. They came under intense scrutiny by research scientists who investigated their loss of ejaculatory ability and/or physical sensation in their genital area. Operating from a medical model—which emphasizes function over other aspects of the person—these researchers' initial concern was with disabled World War II veterans. In retrospect, this obsession with sexual and reproductive function also seems part of a larger cultural anxiety that views any lessening of penile potency as a diminishment of masculinity. This same anxiety is likely related to the phenomenal sales of the impotency drug Viagra among middle and older adult males. This early research largely ignored women, and completely ignored racial and sexual minorities, reflecting that white, heterosexual masculinity was prioritized.

In the past, medical experts have routinely sterilized people with developmental disabilities—and as recently as the early 1970s, disabled people have reported unwanted sterilization. A man whom I interviewed explained that at age twenty-five he underwent a bladder operation but was not told by his physician that one of the outcomes would be loss of ability to ejaculate outside of his body. Instead sperm would be deposited in his bladder. As a young teenager this same man, after having undergone surgery on an undescended testicle, reported that an attending nurse said, "Why did they bother?" While blatant rights violations such as the first example are more infrequent today, the eugenics policies of the past often take more subtle forms such as inherent biases against impairment in genetic and abortion counseling of parents to be.

Because medicine has emphasized correcting deficiencies, it is questionable whether adequate attention has been given to disabled people's capacity for sexual pleasure and reproduction. It is still not unusual for disabled people to report that during physical exams they are not asked any questions about sexuality by their physicians, which is not the case for most non-disabled people. Medical-model research that focuses exclusively on sexual function goes hand in hand with the power and authority medicine wields in disabled people's everyday sexual lives.

Normative understandings of how the body is supposed to function underlie medical diagnoses, treatments, and even rehabilitation and any deviations are targeted for correction. In the case of disease, the medical model is appropriate in order for the patient to "get better." However, impairments are usually permanent and are better understood as bodily variations rather than "deviations." In my own research most of the men I interviewed had reached maturity with poor body images. The majority had a history of medical procedures, surgeries, and rehabilitation therapies, which were aimed at correcting and normalizing their bodies, often to no avail. This medical framing of their bodies as deviant, not only negatively influenced these men's sense of their bodies, but also negatively affected their sexual selves. One of the men I talked to, who had experienced various medical interventions lamented:

> My body image comes directly in my face when I'm dealing in some kind of relationship with a woman. It comes up a lot . . . once again I put pressure on myself. . . . I would say how can she like me with my weird-ass fucking body and the way I walk?

For some disabled people medicine's authority has been diminished by the Disability Rights Movement's success in separating biological impairment from disabling socio-cultural attitudes and practices. On the surface, this distinction between "impairment" and "disability" appears to limit medical authority by focusing clinical attention upon impairment. Disabled people are, in turn, empowered to protest against overt prejudice and oppression in their day to day lives. Disabled people can, it seems, "put medicine in its proper place!" However, upon closer inspection a focus on impairment cannot be easily restricted to disabled people's encounters with physicians and the medical system. A fundamental medical bias that attempts to impose norms upon bodily functions remains unchanged and this influences cultural values and attitudes toward disabled people. Medicine has helped to create and maintain a worship of the "body beautiful" as a cultural imperative. It is a moral edict that exerts tremendous influence on disabled people's body images and sexual selves—as it also impacts many non-disabled people's perceptions of disabled people's sexual desirability.

The emergence of the Disability Rights Movement in the 1970s was a major impetus for challenging the medical model's dominance in understanding disability. This critique was only weakly extended in the case of disability and sexuality research and practitioner interventions. In the late 1970s and early 1980s there was a brief time when disability and sexuality seemed primed to move out from under medical dominance. A disability and sexuality unit at the University of California, San Francisco, which incorporated a social understanding of disability and sexuality issues, was one example of progress in this direction. While some of this work criticized the asexual social attitudes and cultural prejudices directed toward disabled people, and focused on educating professionals who worked with disabled people, a politically charged critique was never sustained. Were it not for a lack of funding during the Reagan years, a political understanding of disability and sexuality might have grown.

In the early 1980s through the mid-1990s, a few advocates attempted to put sexuality on the political and research agendas of the Disability Rights Movement. People such as the late Barbara Waxman and Harlan Hahn, a disabled political scientist, railed against a pronounced lack of social and political analysis on these issues. However, as Waxman has suggested, the Disability Rights Movement as a whole has focused on what they saw as more important access issues such as architectural, transportation, and employment barriers and neglected the more difficult challenge of changing values and attitudes, which underlie much of the sexual oppression of disabled people.

The publication in 1996 of *The Sexual Politics of Disability: Untold Desires* was a major turning point in the debate about disability and sexuality. This critical study conducted in the United Kingdom by Tom Shakespeare, Kath Gillespie-Sells, and Dominic Davies, put sexuality squarely on the political map of the Disability Rights Movement. The authors argue that research on disability and sexuality is still predominately conducted by professionals from medical, psychological, and sexological backgrounds. But this medical and clinical focus has not been sufficiently challenged by disability rights advocates and disability studies scholars. The researchers contend that, "both academics and campaigners have de-prioritized sex and love." The work by Shakespeare, *et al.* is the first systematic study of disability and sexuality that has prioritized the relatively simple goal of discovering what disabled people think and feel about their sexuality. The book chronicles both the sexual oppression encountered by disabled people, as well as the more positive sexual experiences of disabled people. *The Sexual Politics of Disability* has the distinction of having galvanized disability rights activists and disability studies scholars. The subject of disability and sexuality no longer appears to be "fluff" that can wait until after other obstacles to disabled people's rights have been abolished.

Disability and sexuality conferences, a spate of new politically charged writing on sexual oppressions and disabled people's sexual rights, and a lively disability and sexuality listserv all attest to a burgeoning interest in these issues. It has taken a long time but disabled people's sexuality has finally become a central item on the agenda of the Disability Rights Movement and academic disability studies. Progress in transforming disabled people's sexual status and enhancing their sexual well-being will depend on a range of research and advocacy strategies including the framing of issues in terms of sexual rights, the broad public dissemination of disability and sexuality research findings, advocate and activist pressure on media and policymakers, and the self-promotion by disabled people of positive models of their sexuality. Hopefully, increased academic and activist attention to critical disability and sexuality issues coupled with strategies such as these will result in positive changes in public perception of disabled people's sexuality; for starters, replacing the myth of disabled people's asexuality with the more accurate understanding that "of course, they can do that!"

38 Pity dates and the paralyzed playa

The dating scene after spinal cord injury

Tre Trefethen

The BBC talks out their blow hole

A couple of years ago when I was visiting the UK, I caught part of an arts program on the BBC that had two guys squabbling about David Cronenberg's film *Crash*. If you haven't heard of that film, it's about people who get sexual thrills from car accidents. This might seem like a farfetched fetish unless, like I do, you happen to live in San Francisco, where no sexual practice is considered arcane. This was provincial London, however, and one noisy guy in particular was put off by the female lead because she wore a brace. His premise was that the movie was implausible because disabled people have more to worry about than sex, "and it is rather troublesome to think of them in this context." Sigh.

Broken backed Barney Gumble

From a social and sexual standpoint, probably the most frustrating part about break-ing my back was having to endure people in the media making simpleminded pronouncements like that one. Not to generalize, but most of the disabled people I know are obsessed with sex and relationships, probably even more so than the average, nondisabled person, such as pasty film reviewers with bad teeth who work for the BBC. If my own case is an example, in the first years after my accident, everything in my life was about sex. Thoughts like: Would I ever have it again? Would it ever be good? Would anyone love me as I had become? Or barring love, could I at least get a little action without having to pay for it? Sex, sex, sex. It was an all consuming obsession. On the verge of death I would have faded away looking down a nurse's shirt thinking, "Nice tiiiiiiii......ts."

I use a wheelchair and everyone with an obvious impairment like that is lumped into the overarching category, "disabled." People with spinal cord injury, though, are treated as special cases since we provide great human interest stories: there is the sudden loss of many things generally thought of as defining existence. This makes us versatile since we can be either tragic or inspirational, depending on the programming needs, which endears us to the media. Our situation is generally described using a fixed vocabulary of tidy clichés, such as "wheelchair bound" or "paralyzed from the waist down," and these terms strum on familiar cords that produce an emotion unburdened by the exigencies of reality. I get out of bed in the morning and I am the never-say-die hero; I can't feel my cock, I am the tragic eunuch.

It was no wonder, then, that at every party or bar I went to right after my injury I was typecast as the designated neuter. There seemed to be an "Impotent: Flirt with Impunity" sign on my back that told women it was safe to chat with the guy in the wheelchair; there was no danger of me hitting on them. I was inoffensive, harmless, the cute disabled guy. How could their boyfriends object? And guys could relax around me, too, since I wasn't going to compete with them for female attention. I was like the friendly sidekick. Barney Gumble in a wheelchair.

Secret stud

After a few months of this, I began to understand that it was simply a reality that my stature, both physically and psychically, had been diminished by my paralysis, even among my closest friends. For instance, I used to be six feet tall, but I am now something like 3′10″ with my tires pumped. And there's the lack of sensation thing; if you can't feel your cock, people wonder what is the point of having sex? And can you even call it sex? Howard Stern says he would rather be dead than have that happen—that is how incomplete, how bereft of meaning life is without penile sensation. People only see the heroic side of spinal cord injury when we are doing something physical. When they first meet us what they see is always the tragedy.

There are only three ways for a single guy to deal with such a sudden diminution: he could become bitter and sit in his room all day; he could don a zen-like acceptance that he is fated by the stars to live alone; or he could deny it by trying to prove to everyone that everything is just like before. In my own coming to grips with paralysis, the first two methods were out of the question. My libido had survived my accident so I was as horny as ever. There was no way I was going to return to the celibacy of youth if I could possibly beg, borrow, or steal even a semblance of a real sexual encounter.

It was a kind of cross between Maslow and the Twilight Zone that women no longer considered me a commodity, that they didn't even ignore me as an equal in public any more. Even now most women fix me with absent, though benevolent, smiles as they pass by, or chit chat over my head with their friends when I take an elevator. My reaction to this was that I went overboard to demonstrate to everyone how, despite appearances and popular belief, I was a stud.

Blunderbuss Technique, pity dates, and rope-a-dope dating

The first obstacle to proving my virility was overcoming my eunuch status. I figured that most women I knew already established me as nondate material since they had seen my fall from star to humble supporting role. Therefore, I developed what I called the Blunderbuss Technique™, wherein I would ask out as many women as possible. The idea was that, with such a wide spray of propositions, I would hit the mark with some of them and I would get a date.

Of course, this technique by its very nature precludes a hundred percent success, and I knew that the chances were that the woman would refuse; after all, I was living in Vermont at the time, a state where wheelchairs are even scarcer than non-Caucasians. And, too, agreeing to go out does not necessarily constitute a sexual interest. A woman might say "yes" for any number of reasons that may not have been flattering to my ego. Guys in wheelchairs have to be constantly wary of possible humiliation. The way she agrees is the first clue. On the continuum of enthusiasm between "YES!" and "NO!"

the "Pity Date" will be located at ". . . ok", just before the negative, and it is a curse for disabled men, worse than outright refusal.

She says ". . . ok" but when you are out with her, you discover from subtle hints that she only agreed to come because she just feels bad for you, the poor friendly guy in the wheelchair. Rejecting you outright would not mesh with her definition of herself as a politically correct person. Such an evening is not a real date-date, it is a sort of penance she has to endure for being a good and caring person. Women like this, I decided, were to be avoided at all costs.

To forestall other defensive-dating maneuvers, I discovered it was essential to feign a strictly platonic interest and give the impression that this would be just a casual soirée. The best venue in such circumstances was to have dinner at an upscale restaurant. Not only would the place impress, but the woman was seated and, when we were both at that level, I was like any other guy. Even the nice girls who had never thought of me as other than a cute little wheelchair guy would be surprised and gratified that they were sitting across from an actual man. It was a kind of sleight of hand. A feint. Rope-a-dope dating.

The Internet: perpetual ladies' night

Once when we were playing bridge, my grandmother warned me not to shuffle the cards so much or they would end up right back where they started. If the Blunderbuss Technique™ proved successful when I was living in Vermont, it really took off when I moved to San Francisco and there were more women in the deck. Eventually, though, there was a limitation on the number of new women I could meet. That's when I discovered Internet dating.

The Internet is a boon and a bane to disabled people. In one sense, too many disabled people become Internet addicts to the exclusion of getting out in the world and really living. But it also opens up vast horizons, especially for those in rural areas who have no contact with the outside world. Obviously, given the outsider position many of us have in society, it is lonely and isolating for many disabled people. Most don't have the support structure I had, and most don't live in communities that readily accept their difference, so they are forced to be introverts. The Internet works as an equalizer since the person with whom you are communicating cannot see you, can only imagine you based on what you tell them about yourself, and so does not associate you with the clichés and the biases created by the media.

I discovered that it was unwise to tell women I met on the Internet that I use a wheelchair until after we had chatted and they had established a solid idea of me as a man. The idea of a wheelchair is not exactly a chick magnet. After all, paralysis is never going to be a cool thing. No one sane is going to emulate us. And besides, it is perpetual ladies' night on these dating sites and very few self-respecting females would make a wheelchair guy her first pick. So I would send them a couple pictures of myself from the chest up and then, once I had established that I was a regular guy and they showed an interest in meeting, I would send them a couple of me in my chair with the remark that, if they weren't interested after seeing the picture, I understood and no hard feelings. Some I never heard back from, but other women thought of my "confession" as a sign of intimacy, as if I were opening up and revealing a painful truth about myself, and they would agree to go out with me, even if just as a friend. In some weird way, it established me as a "sensitive male." And in some ways, my paralysis was a liberating factor between us. After all, I probably wasn't going to assault them, and if I did, they could no doubt run away, climb a tree, or walk up a few steps to escape me. The fact that I did not ejaculate also made sex with me "safer," at least from a pregnancy standpoint.

All systems go and the two date limit

The paralyzed guy's reaction to society's belief that he is less of a man is to pretend like everything is working in perfect order—so there are several women I was with who never did understand that my penis had no sensation. Even if I had explained this to them, they couldn't reconcile the truth with my Viagra-induced erection, assuming that they had somehow managed to create in me a natural erection. The real reason for this misunderstanding is that I never let on that I had taken the drug. I was like Ray Milland in *The Lost Weekend*, hiding little blue pills around my place so that I could secretly take a little pick-me-up if the situation warranted.

My lack of penile sensation made it so that my focus was not on my own ejaculatory needs and I could concentrate on their pleasure. It wasn't an unselfish giving, though, just the opposite. My purpose was to make love in the strictest sense: to make women love me, or at least to become infatuated with me. I didn't analyze why I was doing this, though. I knew I had something that attracted a certain type of woman to me with first blush; I projected an air of confidence people don't usually associate with the disabled. I had subverted their defenses against men and I was dedicated to their pleasure. In my mind, I did not have anything more than a surface attraction to offer and, if they eventually saw beneath the surface, they would see the realities of my life, the wheelchair and the worries, and be repulsed. After a couple of dates, it felt like the odds were that I would do something to disgust them. I don't mean the stuff you can laugh off, like peeing on a date or causing coitus interruptus by going on a farting jag, but the serious realities of my existence, the exigencies of being a human with no control of body functions. And then she could say to you, you know what, you're a great guy and don't get me wrong, but I would just like to be friends with you. Better by far, I reasoned, was to just hit it and quit it, leaving my mark so that, years from now, they might look back on our time together with regret that I had gotten away. Or at the very least, it was better that they disliked me as a playa, that they actively reviled me, rather than to have them discover the ugly secrets of my real life.

And besides, if you get too close and somehow you have managed to defer the embarrassment or she can laugh when you piss on her, there will come a time when her inability to give you an orgasm begins to pall and she asks, "What can I do to make you feel good?"

The meaning of sex

It's next to impossible to convince a doubtful sensate person that sex without sensation is anything other than a waste of time, but that's not my purpose here. You accept that a paralyzed person is a sexual being or you, like Howard Stern, can't fathom the idea that sex without orgasm can still be fantastic and no amount of talking will convince you otherwise. I can just say that during those early years of my paralysis, I found erogenous zones I didn't know I had. My desires, my fantasies, my ideals of what a woman should look like, all of these became less restrictive than they were before and my enjoyment expanded to all of my senses, not just the enjoyable, but short-lived finale.

Of course, that may sound like I am in denial or trying to play down my losses. After all, if we men with spinal cord injury aren't being portrayed as geldings, we are often striking pre-emptive poses to fend off people patting us on the head, talking down to us like children, or dismissing us entirely. When we get the chance to tell our own stories, you will frequently see us smiling and waving as if everything is just as it always was, or giving a secret wink and a nod to insinuate that we have it even better than before.

But the truth is I do have it better than I did. What happened was that somehow during my sexual peregrinations, a specific woman managed to subvert all my defenses and we realized we love each other. With her it is a totality of sex, the actual physical sharing of the act, but also the emotion of loving someone and the realization that I am loved for who I am despite my limitations and weaknesses. We share a hope and a faith that some day either I will learn some other method than genital stimulation to have orgasms or that future advances will cure my paralysis. In the meantime, our sex is as exciting and as pleasurable as anyone, able-bodied or not, could hope for.

39 Heterosexual and bisexual S/M

Cultural formations

Kathy Sisson

It's hard to believe sadomasochism once hid underground. One has only to pick up a magazine or turn on HBO to observe that the cultural visibility of sadomasochism (S/M) has increased dramatically in the past three decades. Sadomasochistic images appear in fashion and in advertising campaigns. S/M themes punctuate popular books, movies such as 2002's *Secretary* and music such as Madonna's 1992 album *Erotica*. Internet sites with explicit S/M content have proliferated, and books "explaining" S/M to potential participants can be found in the sexuality section of many major bookstores.

The 1990 Kinsey Institute New Report on Sex estimates that, at least occasionally, 5 to 10 percent of the population engages in S/M behavior such as spanking, restraining, or blindfolding. Therefore, using even the most conservative research estimates, millions of individuals in the United States are likely to engage in S/M interactions.

The recent and rapid proliferation of S/M iconography and practice suggests that S/M is a unique reflection of contemporary Western culture. Several cultural theorists claim that late twentieth-century social developments have created mainstream consumers who are receptive to avant-garde representations of transgression, power, sexuality, and risk. In her 1993 essay Anne McClintock writes that S/M sexuality is uniquely suited to our postmodern society because it illustrates the social construction of power, gender roles, identity, and eroticism. After the sexual revolution in the United States and Europe, and in an era when high reproductive rates are less necessary to national economies because of technological innovations, sexual encounters have become easily arranged. They may not, though, have the novelty, uncertainty, and tension that often lent drama to sexual interactions in the past when sex was less readily available for many people. In this context, Foucault described S/M as a power game to heighten sexual intensity.

S/M's apparent increase in popularity in the United States may also be simply the most recent manifestation of an erotic style that predates the use of terminology such as "sadomasochism." Language is tricky in this case because the terms "sadism" and "masochism" only entered the lexicon in 1886 in Krafft-Ebing's *Psychopathia Sexualis*, and "sadomasochism" debuted in 1905 in Freud's *Three Contributions to the Theory of Sex*. Therefore, while we cannot describe behaviors occurring prior to these dates by the term "S/M," abundant evidence suggests that behaviors that are similar to contemporary S/M practices have occurred throughout history.

S/M-type interactions have evolved over time, from isolated instances of individuals seeking to satisfy their particular sexual desire to today's highly visible, nascent S/M culture. These erotic practices and ideals—encompassing a wide range of consensual, interpersonal interactions, from extreme physical sensation to fantasy, and involving eroticized power exchange—have gone through several stages of cultural development.

Examples of isolated individuals combining pain and/or dominance with sexual arousal may date as far back as the Ice Age and at least to antiquity. In *The Prehistory of Sex*, published in 1996, Timothy Taylor describes Venus figurines with bound hands and breasts, estimated to be 25,000 years old. Taylor speculates that these figurines may embody "themes of objectification and possession." Eva Keuls provides photographs of fifth century BCE Grecian vases that depict S/M-like interactions between clients and prostitutes in *Reign of the Phallus*, published in 1985. The *Kama Sutra* (450 CE) discusses sexual biting, pinching, and scratching. Ancient Greek and Roman authors, including Aristotle, Ovid, Petronius, and Lucian, mention various S/M-type interactions in their writings, and several sources from the Middle Ages, such as Pico della Mirandola's *Disputationes Adversus Astrologiam Divinatricem* (1496) and Otto Burnfels' *Onomasticon* (1534), clearly describe individuals who obtained sexual stimulation from whipping.

In the seventeenth, eighteenth, and nineteenth centuries, the second stage in S/M's cultural development emerged as individuals began to increasingly make public their own or others' S/M-type interests. In the seventeenth century, physicians and prostitutes described flagellation as a remedy for erectile dysfunction. S/M-type themes laced popular fictional works such as *The Presbyterian Lash*, *The Virtuoso*, and *Venice Preserv'd*. In the eighteenth century the Marquis de Sade penned his infamous novels and essays, Rousseau wrote about his masochistic predilections in his Confessions, and brothels specializing in flagellation began to appear in major European cities.

These trends expanded into the nineteenth century. Industrialization brought a number of social developments—dramatized power relations, increased privacy, anonymity, leisure time, consumerism, urbanization, and secularization—which promoted particular concepts of sexuality. These social developments also facilitated the public visibility of S/M-type behaviors and increasing numbers of practitioners. Specialized brothels flourished in the United States and Europe and S/M-type themes became more common in popular fiction. Perhaps most importantly, at the century's end the German physician Krafft-Ebing placed S/M behavior squarely into cultural consciousness with the publication of *Psychopathia Sexualis*. His popular typology conferred a name, etiology, and pathology on erotic behaviors and desires that had been considered unremarkable or, at best, medical curiosities.

These nineteenth-century developments fostered the next juncture in S/M's cultural evolution—the formation of practitioner networks and communities. According to Robert Bienvenu, author of a forthcoming book, the modern S/M phenomenon can be traced directly to the early twentieth century, when individual practitioners convened in local, and eventually national and international, networks. S/M moved from public brothels into private spaces and the range of S/M behaviors dramatically expanded. S/M equipment became increasingly specialized and elaborate. Preferences for materials used in S/M activities shifted from soft media (fur, satin, velvet) to hard media (leather, rubber, latex). These materials remain integral in contemporary S/M practice.

By the 1940s S/M practitioners in the United States and Europe formed tight-knit communities around S/M-oriented artists, including photographers, artisans, writers, and publishers. Specialized magazines provided opportunities for contact between like-minded individuals across the country and mail order businesses provided access to equipment and materials. Government censorship and prosecution limited the scope of these communities and enterprises until the 1960s. In the late 1940s and 1950s, a discrete, gay male S/M community emerged, embraced unique iconography and practices, and developed quite differently from the heterosexual/bisexual S/M community.

Several developments in the 1960s contributed to heterosexual/bisexual, S/M cultural evolution. First, the Warren Court handed down increasingly liberal obscenity interpretations in *Roth* v. *US* (1957), *Manual Enterprises* v. *Day* (1962) and *Fanny Hill* (1966). These rulings facilitated the growth of the pornography industry and S/M iconography began to appear in popular pornographic movies and "mainstream" pornographic magazines and books, which drove many small, independent erotica producers out of business. Technological advances made S/M equipment and costumes easier to mass produce, further eroding the small erotica producers' role. Finally, haute couture adopted S/M motifs and S/M began to slowly move toward mainstream fashion. The confluence of these developments ultimately led to the emergence of the first modern heterosexual/bisexual, S/M support groups in the United States in the early 1970s.

Throughout the 1970s, 1980s, and 1990s, increasing numbers of S/M support groups and organizations formed on a national and international scale. By the late 1980s many of these organizations wielded sufficient economic, social, and political power to herald the next stage of cultural development—the formation of a social movement. The Internet greatly accelerated this process by making information about S/M accessible to individuals who were unable or unwilling to join established S/M organizations. The Internet provided cybervenues for likeminded individuals to meet and share experiences. Increased communication between practitioners spurred S/M activism, and those involved with S/M social movements continue to focus on ongoing legal issues involving discrimination, obscenity, and consent. Recently, S/M activists have turned their attention to removing the psychiatric diagnoses that pathologize consensual sadomasochism.

In the 1990s S/M moved into the last stage of cultural development as an embryonic, heterosexual/bisexual, S/M culture emerged. A sexual culture, from an anthropological perspective, is a collective system of meanings and practices that emerges from historically specific social and psychological conditions. Contemporary S/M conforms to this model because S/M practitioners organize, identify, and understand their sexual desires and behaviors through shared mechanisms and ideologies. The emergence of S/M groups also coincide with specific, late twentieth-century cultural conditions— namely, acute social upheaval beginning with Vietnam, the Civil Rights movement, and feminism, and extending through postmodern philosophy's rejection of traditional intellectual paradigms.

Contemporary S/M culture reflects both historical and more recent social developments but this does not mean that this new sexual culture is static. As S/M sexual culture becomes further integrated into mainstream culture, it continues to be malleable and subject to internal and external pressures similar to those faced by other stigmatized, emergent sexual cultures.

Will S/M cultures continue to merge with mainstream fashion and eventually be regarded as passé by a public with a short attention span? Will this ultimately lead to certain practitioners rejecting S/M because it no longer reflects a significant transgression of the status quo? Or will S/M retain its distinctive ideology, iconography, and cultural attributes—securing a place as a recognized sexual identity? How S/M continues to evolve in Western culture over the next century will demonstrate as much about mainstream sexualities as it does about alternative sexualities.

40 Ms etiquette and the transgender employee

Is *nothing* private any more?

Jillian Todd Weiss

Gender transition used to be a very private matter. The patient would disappear from his or her hometown and reappear somewhere else, ready for a fresh start with a different gender. The patient was strongly advised to keep the past secret. Those who failed to do so often regretted the severe social disapproval their indiscretions reaped.

Now, however, gender transition commonly occurs in the workplace as law, public relations, and political correctness combine to make society and employers more trans-friendly. Upper management and nameless coworkers know intimate details of the private life of an employee in transition. Even something as personal as who can use what bathroom has become an HR issue.

The bathroom is a flashpoint for conflicting levels of social tolerance. The importance of these strictly private spaces for males and females is taught to us very early in life. The separation of the sexes is a product of the understanding that a person's biological sex determines their psychology, their social role, and their sexuality. Now, we are asked to accept that George can become Christine, contradicting what we have been taught about the gulf between the sexes. Violation of these spaces touches on many pivotal identity issues—privacy of excretory functions, fear of public nudity, our identification with people of the same gender, appropriate sexuality, sexual harassment, and violence against women. The image of a "man in a dress" in the ladies' bathroom (or the men's bathroom) brings up these issues in a visceral way. As an abstract proposition, many are prepared to live and let live. The abstract becomes concrete, however, when we find ourselves standing next to Christine in the bathroom mirror. As a society, we do not tolerate gender ambiguity well.

Is nothing private any more? Some would prefer that issues of sexuality be restricted to the private sphere and kept out of the workplace. Most transgender employees would prefer that as well. However, when gender transition takes place in the workplace, there can be little expectation of complete privacy because it is, by its very nature, a public changing of gender identity. How do we reformulate the balance between what is private and what is public?

There is no easy answer because "privacy" is itself a relative term in modern society. When a worker goes from female to male or vice versa, he or she must give up the notion of a discreet transition. Does that give distant coworkers the right to ask rude questions? Hardly. But management—don't they at least have to know, well, shall we say certain details in order to assign the proper bathroom? And don't coworkers who share the facilities have a right to know who is standing (or sitting) next to them in the lavatory? What *is* the proper business etiquette? What *would* Emily Post say? (I imagine she would be speechless.)

Men's restroom?

One of the factors in this privacy determination is the traditional law of employment, called the "employment at will doctrine." It gives a private employer the right to hire or fire an employee for any reason or no reason at all. Employers also have the right to set the terms and conditions of employment. This rule has been undermined, however, in regard to certain forms of discrimination. Race discrimination became illegal in the United States about forty years ago. The list of protected categories has expanded greatly, and now it is widely considered immoral (though not necessarily illegal) to discriminate on any grounds unrelated to the job. More than a dozen states and well over a hundred local governments have prohibited employers from discriminating on the basis of "gender identity." This does not, however, remove signs from bathroom doors. There is a law, for example, in Minnesota that forbids discrimination against transgender employees. An employee who transitioned from male to female used the women's restroom. The employer objected and effectively terminated the employee. The employee filed a lawsuit, and the Minnesota Supreme Court decided the employee had no discrimination claim based on her transgender status. It ruled that the law was not intended to overturn the "cultural preference" for sex segregated facilities. It did not consider the irony that similar reasoning once justified race segregated facilities.

In its ruling the court unwittingly subordinated another principle that we value highly: medical privacy. We consider it improper (and unlawful) for an employer to ask about the medical history of employees unless there is some bona fide need because of the nature of the job requirements, for example, the vision of airline pilots. Asking an employee in the accounting department about their genitals is probably not a bona fide occupational requirement. And yet, allowing guys into the ladies' room is definitely not an idea whose time has come.

Whole is greater than the sum of its parts

The medical realities of sex reassignment surgery are important here. There is a popular idea that "sex change surgery" transforms a hypermasculine Arnold Schwarzenegger into a super-feminine Nicole Kidman, or vice versa. There is, however, no such thing. Instead, there are several dozen medical treatments and surgical procedures that can be involved in sex reassignment. These change various primary and secondary sexual characteristics. The choice of procedures varies greatly and may depend on medical and financial health. While many trans people undergo surgery that creates genitals of the opposite sex, most do not. Fewer female-to-male transsexuals have full phalloplasty, as genital surgery for female-to-male transsexuals is much more expensive and the results are often less than convincing. Genital surgery also does not change one's public appearance or the ability to pass as the opposite sex—that's mostly a matter of dress and grooming. The level of coworker comfort usually relates to the level of visible gender ambiguity—how well the transgender person blends into their chosen sex. Mental health professionals use an eight-point test to discuss gender[1] and often talk about gender being a "social construction" rather than a biological one. Thus, a simple surgical requirement doesn't pass muster.

As a consultant to large employers on this issue, I have found that while initially, managers often zero in on medical and legal issues, this focus rarely provides satisfactory answers. No sane employer wants to become part of the transgender employee's medical team or litigate the complex issues of gender transition. The imposition of a surgical requirement by a company may pose legal problems with the typical health insurance exclusion for transsexual surgery. At the same time, a business decision *must* be made about sensitive issues such as bathroom usage. The decision should, of course, respect the transgender employee, while also accounting for the concerns of coworkers. The lack of social consensus about gender transition means that there can be no hard and fast rules. Each case must be approached on its own merits. However, while a case-by-case approach sounds reasonable, it can turn into arbitrary and capricious decision making that unfairly burdens trans employees. This is not good for employers if there is future litigation. There are, however, several general criteria that can be used to point managers in the right direction. For example, managers may consider the number of bathrooms within reasonable walking distance, the availability of single use or lockable bathrooms, the length of the trans employee's transition, and the comfort level of trans employees and coworkers. One possible option: an employer could host an information session for coworkers to notify them of company policy and expected norms of conduct, announcing that Jane will henceforth use the third-floor restroom. This permits uncomfortable coworkers to use another restroom. Generally, such coworkers get over it after a while, but forcing ideas upon them can cause bad feelings and litigation.

The etiquette of modern business is tricky—we want employers to "do the right thing," but figuring out the "right thing" is often confusing. There is an increasing occurrence of workplace gender transitions. It was unknown in 1952, when George Jorgensen's transition to Christine hit the nation's headlines. My research with large employers shows that the current prevalence in large organizations is probably up to 0.01 percent. This is a small number, but it means that in a corporation of 10,000 there is probably one person who has transitioned on the job. The increasing acceptance of gender transition in society means that many employers, particularly large ones, will likely face such decisions at some time in the near future.

Transgender employees who transition in the workplace can not expect others to ignore the change, for it is by nature a public event. At the same time, privacy and dignity have their place even in public events. From a sound business policy viewpoint, the public nature of the event requires reasonable accommodation and clear policy to set the norms of corporate behavior, but private details of the transition should remain private. Like any business decision, workplace transition rules are informed by medical and legal opinions, but primarily based on business considerations of workplace harmony and the increased productivity and profit that results. Not even Emily Post would disagree with that, I am sure.

Note

1   See Brown, Mildred L., and Rounsley, Chloe Ann. 1996. *True Selves: For Families, Friends, Coworkers and Helping Professionals.* Jossey-Bass, San Francisco, CA, p. 20. Brown and Rounsley assert that there are at least eight factors to be considered in determining gender, five biological and three social and psychological. "The biological determinants are chromosomes, hormones, gonads (glands that produce sex hormones), internal sexual and reproductive organs and external sex organs. The social and psychological determinants are gender of rearing, gender role, and gender identity." While it is true that the DSM mentions four factors to be considered in making a diagnosis of "gender identity disorder," I am speaking here about a determination of "gender," not "gender identity disorder." In addition, even under the DSM, one must also consider the physical differential factors to be used in excluding a diagnosis of intersex.

41 At the Cesar Chavez Institute

Bridging academic research and community empowerment

Joyce Nishioka

Rafael Diaz works on the corner of 16th and Mission, an area of San Francisco populated with underprivileged immigrants and down-and-out natives, a place with more than its share of wheelchairs and despair, where heroin dealers deal and homeless addicts come to get their fix. In his office on the third floor of a lowrise building, Diaz recalls the experiences that compelled him to work for social justice. In the early 1990s he was a tenured professor at Stanford, a "rising star," he says. At the same time, many of his friends were dying from AIDS. Nearly every weekend he would descend from the ivory tower and head north to San Francisco for yet another memorial. "This was the reality of life," he explains.

Searching for work with a more direct impact on people, Diaz resigned from Stanford in the early 1990s and enrolled in a post-doctorate epidemiology program at the University of California, San Francisco. Through studying gay Latino men, he came to grasp the value of people's real life experiences. Theorizing about social problems without first collaborating with those affected no longer made sense to him. That conviction led him to the streets of San Francisco's Mission District, where, with microphone in hand, he conducted interviews with gay and bisexual Latino men at risk for HIV infection. His research culminated with the publication of his book *Latino Gay Men and HIV: Culture, Sexuality and Risk Behavior*, a seminal work exploring the diversity of gay life in the backdrop of the AIDS epidemic.

Today, Diaz's socially engaged approach to scholarship is the foundation of San Francisco State University's Cesar Chavez Institute (CCI), where he is the director. Acting as a bridge between academic research and the community empowerment, the institute produces studies documenting the impact of social oppression on the health and well-being of minority communities—while affirming the strength and resiliency of the underprivileged and underserved. The lineage of Diaz's philosophy can be traced back to Paulo Freire's theory of critical consciousness. Freire, a Brazilian educationalist who wrote *Pedagogy of the Oppressed*, viewed learning as an act of freedom. Through education and dialogue, people could gain the knowledge and power needed to expand their social capital and improve their communities.

Hermanos de Luna y Sol (Brothers of the Moon and Sun) embodies Diaz's community-approached research and Freire's philosophy. The nonprofit program, housed three blocks from the Cesar Chavez Institute at Mission Neighborhood Health Center, targets gay and bisexual men, as well as transgender women, among the district's Latino immigrant community.

There, Project Coordinator Héctor Ceballos refrains from lecturing to participants. Instead he encourages them to share their experiences and learn from each other. They examine the history of their oppression and then analyze their behaviors. They look at situations where they were vulnerable and eventually, become empowered to use better self-judgment.

And they talk with brazen honesty. Even when discussing serious topics, they feel comfortable enough to chime in and challenge each other while managing to laugh at themselves and each other. Ceballos recalls one man who in describing an encounter quipped, "I was trying to convince him to wear a condom—and on top of that his dick was so enormous that it was not going anywhere!" Ceballos says, "These men and women are resilient and have overcome so much, yet they are convivial. They come here and their experiences are validated."

Ceballos's work is a crucial part of the attempt to stem the AIDS epidemic among Latinos. Nationwide, this group makes up about 13 percent of the US population but accounts for 18 percent of all AIDS cases reported and 20 percent of diagnoses made in 2002. Latino men who have sex with men (MSM) face even grimmer statistics. A 2002 study by University of California's AIDS Research Program found more than 35 percent of young gay and bisexual Latino men in the border town of San Diego were infected with HIV.

So far, some 1,200 people, mostly Mexican immigrants, have participated in the *Hermanos de Luna y Sol*. Most of them live on the outskirts of the mainstream. In the United States they struggle because of language barriers and limited job opportunities, but at the same time, discover newfound freedom to express their sexuality. "That is very alluring," Ceballos says. "In Mexico many gay men idealize white men. They come here and can have them. It is easy to have sex; guys want them; they are exoticized." Too often, though, they do not have the confidence or skills to negotiate safe sex:

> In Latino culture you do not talk about sex, especially not gay sex. I find that many of the men new to the program will use euphemisms to allude to sex—for example, "We did what we had to do and then left." We encourage them to be graphic, to use whatever vocabulary they need to communicate with their sexual partners.

Diaz acts as *Hermanos de Luna y Sol's* program evaluator. The discrimination many gay and bisexual Latino men are confronted with—mainly racism, poverty, and homophobia—results in social isolation and psychological distress, he explains. Such distress makes them vulnerable to risky behavior: they may be less able to negotiate safe sex because of an enhanced fear of rejection or unequal power sharing in the relationship; they may use sex and/or drugs to relieve their distress. Social isolation traps them in this destructive cycle. "Sexual risk behavior is predicted by discrimination. Factors that help moderate the situation may be gaining family acceptance, having a sense of community with friends and social networks, or participating in social activism," Diaz says.

More work to be done

One of Cesar Chavez Institute's five current onsite projects is the Family Acceptance Program, directed by Caitlin Ryan. Like all of the work at the Institute, it is a good example of the process of socially-engaged scholarship.

The Family Acceptance Program was created in 2002, based on an earlier finding that there was only one program in California to help LGBT youth engaged families.

"Families are important but most programs get away from the family, in a sense protect young people from their families," Diaz says. "We wanted to see if family acceptance could actually protect youth." In the first phase of the project, researchers conducted in-depth interviews with underserved LGBT youth and their families throughout California, in English and Spanish. They included immigrant families, as well as rural and resource-poor families. Some of the young people were in foster care. Researchers then converted the interviews into a survey that they administered to twenty-one to twenty-five-year-old gay men and lesbians. The survey consisted of experiential questions, Diaz says, such as: "Did your parents connect you to LGBT resources?" "Did your parents express homophobia or anger when you came out?" "Did your parents allow your LGBT friends into the house?" "Did your parents support how you looked and how you dressed?"

"The questions were asked retroactively, so that from the data we could find out which parental actions are helpful and which are risky. It is all based on the voices of the community," he says. The Family Acceptance Program is now in the stage of developing evidence-based training and intervention materials. "It may be that taking your child to PRIDE is not helpful, but helping them find role models who are successful sexual minorities with jobs and regular lives, is. Practitioners need to know this and involve the family." Throughout the process the community—advocates, health workers, teachers, youth—was involved, helping to recruit interviewees, discussing interview data, and interpreting survey results.

Diaz is continuing his own research. Currently, he is studying drug use among Latino gay and bisexual men and transgender women, testing his hypothesis that community involvement tempers the negative effects of poverty, racism, and homophobia. Though Diaz is himself a gay, Latino man, he says, "I'm not studying myself." His upper-middle-class family fled Cuba when he was eleven and settled in Venezuela. At twenty-two he came to the United States to study social work at NYU, and then went to Yale to earn his doctorate in psychology. Despite his privileged upbringing, he says with some reserve, "My family did suffer as immigrants; my parents were Cuban exiles coming to a new country trying to gain acceptance. Yes, I have experienced homophobia too. My own wounds fuel my passion and activism."

42 My intersex journey

From awkward teenager to human rights activist

David Cameron

At fourteen I hadn't developed like other boys and was often teased for having very small testicles. They often stayed up inside of me. It was an awkward time for me as I was very tall and slender. I was a self-conscious, sensitive, and emotional kid. My mother, concerned about my lack of development, took me to the family doctor for an examination. Without any tests, he assured her that I would grow up "normal" and be able to have children.

But by my early twenties I developed breasts and had cellulite-type hairless fatty tissue over most of my body. I had gender identity issues and generally was sexually attracted to men. In college after taking interest tests, I was told that my interests were "too feminine." My father used to tell me, "You are just like your mother." I often felt wedged between genders and had to deal with my difference alone.

I remembered from high school biology that "giants" were usually sterile. I wondered if I might be, too, since I was 6' 10". In my late twenties I went to an infertility clinic to investigate. *I was shocked by the diagnosis!*

The term "intersex" is still an enigma to many people. I was introduced to the term in 1995, when I went to my first intersex support group led by Cheryl Chase, the founder of the Intersex Society of North America (ISNA). There, it was explained that intersex was a variation in sexual anatomy as compared to what one might consider standard "male" and "female."

Intersex is an umbrella term. It could be a large clitoris that doctors decide needs to be trimmed down, or a micropenis that physicians examine to determine if it is big enough for heterosexual sex. Many intersex people have standard XX (female) and XY (male) sex chromosomes while others do not. In Androgen Insensitivity Syndrome (AIS), XY children's genitals feminize without any internal female sex organs and, depending on the person, individual gender identity can vary. Those with Turner's Syndrome have XO chromosomes (a missing X chromosome). Those with the endocrine and chromosomal variation called Klinefelter's Syndrome, which occurs in about one out of every 500 to 1,000 "male" births, have XXY sex chromosomes.

After extensive examinations and tests, I was told that I had Klinefelter's Syndrome. I was informed that I was sterile and that my tiny testicles only produced 10 percent of the testosterone levels of "normal males."

Medicalizing intersex

Without any emotional counseling I was advised to immediately start testosterone replacement therapy. I was told that my sex drive would increase, I would gain weight and my shoulders would broaden, and that I would have to inject myself with 300mg of testosterone every two weeks for life. Medical journals called my condition "feminized" male.

Doctors offered breast reduction surgery and testicular implants but I refused. My gender identity was never discussed. And they didn't tell me that I was about to go through puberty again *with a vengeance* . . . in my thirties. It was fun to be a teenager again. I wasn't particularly horny the first time I went through puberty. This time was different. I grew a beard, got very hairy everywhere and started to go bald. I liked the beard but not the other side effects, including prostate enlargement.

Within five years, my small prostate had grown so large that I had to take medication to urinate. When injecting testosterone I experienced a sexual energy surge within a short time. I was not used to this and became extremely sexually active. And then I contracted HIV. As a result of the testosterone, my body changed in ways that altered my sense of self.

In retrospect, after twenty-eight years of injections, I now realize that my body was alright the way it was. I didn't need to change it. My endocrinologist was not God, although I trusted that he knew what was best for me at the time. My sexuality and gender confusion was based on the idea that I was supposed to turn out heterosexual— *not homosexual*. My attraction to men was supposed to be a phase.

In a sense, I was a heterosexual female. I feel that I was rushed into an experience that I wasn't ready for and that my doctor deceived me. Doctors do not have all the correct information on sex, gender, and sexuality diversity. Not everything needs to be pathologized just because it is *different*. I've had to learn to trust my own life experience, not fitting into our "two sex/two genders: Western binary system." I often wonder why I was created, never to reproduce in our family-obsessed culture.

Proud to be me

After that first intersex support group, I learned that, for me, my sense of gender as a "blend" is okay. One's "sex" and "gender" are separate issues. I became Cheryl's first ISNA volunteer and eventually lead its support group. I now speak at many venues where I share my experience of living with an intersex anatomy.

In 1996 Cheryl and I were part of a small panel that informed the San Francisco Human Rights Commission's (HRC's) Lesbian, Gay, Bisexual, and Transgender (LGBT) Advisory Committee of the reality of intersex people. This panel started my journey as an intersex human rights activist. In 2000, I was appointed to the San Francisco Transgender Civil Rights Implementation (SFTGCRI) Task Force as an intersex person. At that time "intersex" was included under the "transgender" umbrella. There is some overlap between the two, but intersex has its own "umbrella" of different anatomical realities.

Through my participation and education of the Task Force, I was able to get intersex separated from the transgender umbrella and put into a category all its own. It was ironic to me that transgender persons who wanted to transition to another sex had to pay out of pocket for those "cosmetic" interventions, while intersex children were covered by their parents' insurance companies as long as their transition occurred before they could give legal consent.

After the conclusion of the SFTGCRI Task Force, I continued to work with the Human Rights Commission Lesbian, Gay, Bisexual, Transgender Advisory Committee on their Gender Identity working group as a community member. We voted to create an Intersex Task Force. The task force worked on creating a public hearing at the request of the Commissioners and this "historic event" was held on May 27, 2004. This was the first time a governmental body in the United States had ever addressed intersex human rights issues! A resolution approved by the San Francisco Board of Supervisors proclaimed October 26, 2004 as the first annual Intersex Awareness Day. A group of intersex activists attended the ceremony at San Francisco City Hall. Emi Koyama, executive director of Intersex Initiative (www.intersexinitiative.org), requested the resolution's adoption on behalf of intersex persons worldwide. Betsy Driver, executive director of Bodies Like Ours (www.bodieslikeours.org), cosponsored the event.

For intersex people, who often travel a painful and long journey to gain acceptance, this was truly a joyous and monumental occasion.

Part 5

The globalization of sexuality

With millions of dollars funneled into HIV/AIDS-prevention campaigns around the world and pornography from the far reaches of the planet available almost instantaneously, with sex tourism in Southeast Asia and panics about sexual slavery in the United States, it is clear that we now live in an age where sexuality, in its many manifestations, has gone global. To think about sexuality—one of the most personal and intimate aspects of our lives—in this way may seem counterintuitive. However, by bringing the personal into a larger political context, the multiple facets of sexuality in our contemporary era come together; we cannot ignore how sexuality is implicated in the large-scale changes occurring around the world.

Considering sexuality in global and transnational frameworks links together sexual rights, health, education, and commodification, along with questions about what counts as morality or social values in different cultural settings. Taking national, historical, and economic differences into account becomes mandatory when we think about sexuality on global terrain. It also demands that we "think outside the box" and evaluate our own assumptions and value systems. Understanding the intimacies of sexuality in global dimensions, we are pushed to question and problematize our own assumptions about what is right and wrong or what we perceive as "natural" regarding sexuality.

Understanding sexuality across human experience

In Western societies there has been a long tradition of studying sexuality from the point of view of biology, medicine, and pathology, and sex as a function in the perpetuation of our species. In addition to biomedical approaches to the study of sexuality, the social sciences and humanities have approached the question of sexuality, in general, in two distinct ways. On the one hand, sexuality has been assessed through the lens of psychoanalysis and Freudian concepts of desire, repression, and sublimation. More recently, following the French theorist Michel Foucault, the study of sexuality has emphasized the "proliferation of discourse" surrounding sexuality. From this vantage point, a critique of the psychoanalytic approach, Freud's "repressive hypothesis," becomes yet another cog in a larger machine that produces "sexuality" as an abstraction in the service of medical, educational, military, and identity projects.

Studies of sexuality outside of the West have sometimes been criticized for exoticizing (or some would say, fetishizing) the sexuality of people in faraway lands. Some academic and popular literatures have tended to emphasize the salacious and shocking aspects of sexual difference found around the world. However, a large body of comparative studies, in anthropology for example, emphasizes a shared continuum of sexual behavior and desire across human experience, from homoerotics in Papua New Guinea to shifting notions of romance across the US/Mexican border. Works such as these maintain that cultural variation accounts for very different manifestations of sexual behavior. Given this history in scholarship, are there ways that we can think about sexuality both within and outside the borders of the United States that neither homogenizes nor exoticizes human sexuality?

Sexuality in the global morality market

By flipping on the television in just about any country in the world, one will find traces of US-styled sexuality, exported through syndicated TV shows, movies, and advertising. Has the advent of global capitalism and the spread of information technologies led to an "Americanization" of sexuality? Are soap opera-styled liaisons or surgically endowed femininity becoming the norm internationally, much like the supposed "Coca-Cola-ization" of culture? Or is the opposite at work, with the United States becoming exposed to alternative conceptions of sexuality from other countries and cultures? Before we can begin to answer this question, we must first ask what exactly is "American sexuality." Is there only one or are there many different and disparate ways of understanding sexuality in the United States and thus around the world? According to recent analyses of sexuality in the world system, we must begin to see sexuality very much like we see the movement of people, commodities, and capital investment in the twenty-first century: circulating.

However, sexuality is not experienced the same everywhere. For instance, there have been very different concepts about what constitutes "homosexuality" in Latin America versus the Middle East or urban North America. Is homosexuality a matter of one's behavior (sexual acts with someone of the same biological sex) or is homosexuality a self-claimed identity, a process of exiting the closet and articulating one's desire and same-sex attraction? "Homosexuality" as a medical term might not even be capable of capturing the diversity of people's experiences, much less designate the significance attributed to these experiences. In a similar vein, the meaning ascribed to prostitution and the "selling" of sexual acts is different in West Africa than it is in Atlanta. How do we then account for different cultural, as well as individual, interpretations of sexual labor in a transnational context?

Sexuality in global perspective involves volatile controversies. The trafficking of women and children for sexual labor—whether forced or voluntary—involves multiple networks, border crossings, and financial transactions. Sexual trafficking also begs the question of what counts as "voluntary" involvement in prostitution. With so many girls and women struggling for a basic existence in many parts of the world, "survival sex" or subsistence prostitution, raises many questions about the commodification of sex, moral responsibility, and the governmental and social structures that have led to these situations. When feminists ally themselves with social conservatives in attempts to eradicate the illicit trade in women and girls in "sexual slavery," we find the politics of morality deeply implicated in contemporary policy debates around sexuality.

Prostitution surrounding military bases is nothing new; it has long been considered by many military planners to be requisite for the rest and relaxation of troops. As military and militia presence is transformed, dislocated from cold war bastions and stationed in newly volatile regions, we must inquire into how this is changing the shape of the sexual world in conflict zones and back at home. Sexual war crimes such as mass rape demand that we account for sexual violence in more troubling and vast dimensions. In these kinds of situations, sexuality cannot be understood as simply a set of negotiated desires between consenting adults. Whether we are talking about UN peacekeepers stationed in African conflict zones, or US military bases abroad, regional militarization and the implications this has for residents are profound on both social and sexual levels.

As we increasingly bring questions of "morality" to bear upon global sexuality, we are at an historic crossroads. How do we begin to formulate a set of universally recognizable and agreed-upon attitudes when social values are so different in diverse cultural contexts? Global debates about female genital surgery or FGS (also called female genital mutilation, circumcision, or "cutting"), for example, have tread upon questions of health, reproduction, pleasure, the status of women, and transnational values, as well as international legal norms. Are these surgeries a violation of human rights? Or are they simply a manifestation of a cultural ethos surrounding women's sexuality? And must the two be diametrically opposed? Huge sums of funding are put toward population control programs, abstinence-oriented sex prevention campaigns, HIV/AIDS reduction strategies, and sexual exploitation abatement. These financial flows of capital and investments in what we might call a "sexual infrastructure," demonstrate how sexual morals and values are deployed by countries that donate large amounts of funding. In turn, we see how sexuality may be changed and assumptions shifted by the kind of outreach that occurs on the ground. In this Part, consider how cultural values and moralities about sexuality in diverse contexts coincide. Ask whether there is a global norm to be established around sexual rights, sexual health, and sexuality education as you consider sexuality on a global scale.

43 Global perspectives on sexual rights

Sonia Corrêa with Cymene Howe

In the international news and in social justice struggles here in the United States, we hear a lot about "human rights." However, many people may not know its history. Human rights principles and discourses of the eighteenth century were revived in the context of the United Nations in response to the Nazi Holocaust. Many countries signed onto these principles, and since then human rights has grown and changed. In the last thirty years we have seen major developments in the ways that governments and non-governmental organizations and advocates have turned to human rights in order to create gender and sexual equality and to protect sexual diversity around the world. Of course the controversies are many. In this conversation, we speak with a leading thinker and activist who has been involved with the struggle for gender and sexual rights, to ask her about the origins of, and possible futures for, sexual rights in the twenty-first century.

Can you tell us about the genesis of human rights and how they have become so central to our contemporary understanding of the world and social justice movements?
SONIA CORRÊA: The history of human rights has been the history of integrating civil and political rights with economic and social rights. It has also been the history of expanding the potential subjects and areas to which human rights can be applied—women, children, black people, indigenous people. This expansion characterizes the modern and contemporary history of human rights. Within this, the very last frontier was sexuality, sexual orientation, and identity. The first time it appeared at the level of intergovernmental negotiations was in the 1994 International Conference on Population and Development in Cairo. The term "sexual rights and reproductive rights" was drafted, though in the end just "reproductive rights" was retained in the final document.

But long before that, we had been struggling with the idea that sexuality is a domain of freedom, as well as one where persons must be protected from inequality and abuse. In the 1960s in the United States, notions of sexual liberation and sexual politics evolved concurrently with the civil rights movements. In Latin America in the late 1970s and 1980s, a similar trend was witnessed in connection to democratization. The road was then open to strongly link sexuality and citizenship rights.

The next step would be the transportation of these struggles to human rights regimes that are not bounded by nation-states. Within that move it is important to underline that until the 1990s the main approach to human rights on a global scale was largely derived from the French and US revolutions, which underscored that citizens must be protected from powerful governments, usually their own. It has taken us two hundred years to acknowledge that human rights abuses are also perpetrated by other agents, not just in the public sphere but also in the private sphere. Still, the notion that human rights abuses are carried out by private agents, particularly in the context of families, is not entirely settled upon, either politically or conceptually.

More specifically, how have sexual rights developed through the United Nations' meetings, conferences and forums of the last twenty years or so?
SONIA CORRÊA: The first reference to gender equality and human rights appears in the Universal Declaration of Human Rights, which was developed in 1948. Article 2 states: "Everyone is entitled to all the rights and freedoms set forth in this Declaration, without distinction of any kind, such as race, color, sex, language, religion, political or other opinion, national or social origin, property, birth or other status." This very clearly spells out that nobody can be discriminated against upon the basis of sex—in this case, "sex" actually refers to gender.

However, as recently as the 1993 World Conference on Human Rights in Vienna, the notion of women's human rights was contested.

The term "sexual rights" appeared for the first time in 1994 in a UN intergovernmental document on the Cairo Program of Action at the International Conference on Population and Development. However, "sexual rights" was not yet a part of an agreed text. At the Fourth World Conference on Women in 1995, the Beijing Declaration finally legitimized the notion of women's human rights in all spheres of life. A definition was adopted of women's human rights in the realm of sexuality, which would become the icon of sexual rights in current global and national debates on the subject. However, a consensus could not be reached on the issue of discrimination based on sexual orientation. The next step was the 2001 World Conference Against Racism, Racial Discrimination, Xenophobia, and Related Intolerance in Durban, South Africa, where a paragraph on discrimination on the basis of sexual orientation was presented but rejected.

The 2003 resolution on human rights and sexual orientation presented by Brazil at a United Nations Human Rights Commission session was the culmination of this process. For the first time a full UN text will explicitly state that sexual orientation is not a justifiable basis for discrimination. If adopted, the resolution would be a critical step for transforming international legislation on the matter. If nothing else, in the current global climate where the voices of Bush and the Vatican on homosexuality gain increasing leverage, the Brazilian Resolution has crucial symbolic value.

Can you describe the importance of the Beijing World Conference on Women in 1995 and Beijing+5 in 2000, as well as other UN conferences, in transforming ideas and legislation around gender and sexual rights?
SONIA CORRÊA: The Beijing conference has to be situated in a larger historical frame. It was not the first conference on women; in fact, it was the fourth. It was preceded by Nairobi in 1985, Copenhagen in 1980, Mexico in 1975, as well as by the adoption in 1979 of the Convention for the Elimination of all Forms of Discrimination Against Women, not yet ratified by the United States.

At the same time, you cannot understand what happened in Beijing and the previous conferences without taking into account what is happening in societies around the world. The outcomes of the conference can not be seen as something floating, abstractly hovering above us. In the last decade, the UN has really opened itself up to listening to civil society, nongovernmental organizations, and advocacy groups. This has been a strategic process to create a new global consensus on relevant issues like women's rights, human rights, and population.

The Beijing conference was particularly relevant because it expressed very power-fully the fact that women's issues were a subject of public concern and discourse in the most diverse societies. The diversity of women present in the Beijing Forum, which was run parallel to the UN conference, was much more evident than in previous conferences.

I was in Nairobi in 1985, and I would say that probably 80 percent of the delegates were men. Very few delegations, particularly from developing countries had women heading the delegations. In 1995, 95 percent of the delegates were women and this was true even of delegations from countries that were openly resistant to notions of gender equality, like Yemen. Even those countries felt embarrassed to send male delegates, which tells you a lot about the changes we saw in just ten years' time.

In terms of content the Beijing Platform for Action was a very ambitious policy document. We were there not just to talk about specific problems of gender inequal-ity; we were addressing human rights, violence, media, health, armed conflicts, and market economies. There was also a more clear understanding of how gender systems and gender inequality are structural dimensions that need to be addressed when you are talking about development projects such as economic structural adjustment pro-grams, the labor market, the environment, safe water, housing initiatives, and disease prevention and reduction.

Each of the UN conferences you have been describing are of course global in scope, drawing from countries around the world and attempting to come to consensus on what are often very controversial and pressing issues. But what role does the United States play, in particular, in these negotiations? Perhaps Beijing provides a good illustration of the dynamics.

SONIA CORRÊA: Frankly, something very big happened in the 1990s at the global level. An incredible, visionary, and forward-looking consensus had been reached in relation to human rights, population, and the environment. The end of the cold war had created promises, a decline in military expenditures, and the possibility of better understanding in the global community. The Clinton administration had a very strong commitment to gender equality and the human rights of women. The US position was often conservative in regard to economic and security issues. But under the pressure of US-based activists and of Southern countries, it showed relative flexibility with respect to economic issues when conflicts between the North ("developed" or "first" world) and the South ("underdeveloped" or "third" world) that surged at the conferences, threatened gender equality and women's human rights.

This changed entirely with the Bush administration. On the most controversial dimensions of women's human rights, which relates to reproduction and sexuality, the Bush administration has been systematically regressive. It is an awkward and seemingly contradictory discourse because, on the one hand, there is much discussion about women in political positions of power in Afghanistan and Iraq, or the argument that one of the objectives for the invasion of Afghanistan was the liberation of women from the Taliban. At the same time, there has been a lack of support for women's human rights in practice.

In the UN process anybody can say, "I don't agree." You can make reservations, declarations, or resolutions. But the United States has also bullied countries. They refer to the amount of money that they are providing. It is very problematic to have a negotiation under those conditions because many of these countries are extremely fragile. It's very hard for a poor country to take a stand when the United States is saying, "If you don't behave, we're going to suspend all the money you're getting."

The so-called Cairo-friendly or Beijing-friendly countries have been very concerned about a global conference for women in 2005 because the political conditions were very, very risky. Even before the current US administration came to power, the Vatican and Islamic countries resisted the Cairo and Beijing conferences. With that combination of forces—and the possibility that a global conference could destroy the consensus built in 1995—there is a lot of concern.

If you were to predict some of the issues the UN will face over the next ten years with regards to its sexual rights efforts, what would you say are the key struggles?
SONIA CORRÊA: A new backlash, now global, is clearly underway, which is largely generated by fundamentalism in various forms: theocracy in Islamic countries and Pentecostal and radical fringes of the Catholic Church in many other countries. In Latin America, for example, we see a growing emphasis on fundamentalist interpretations, not only in relation to gender among religious forces, but also in other realms as it is the case of ethnic and nationalist based movements. All over the world these regressive forces increasingly zero in on sexuality and gender equality as a primary target. This necessarily reflects on global policy arenas.

All of this is taking place at a moment in history when we have extreme inequalities around the world; there are huge numbers of people being integrated into a larger global system, while many others are left outside. Many of the fundamentalist forces are drawing from those on the margins, those who have not been included. Therefore, a prospectively sound human rights agenda—with respect to gender equality and sexuality—must be deeply connected to providing livelihoods. There are groups of women and gays and lesbians who are well integrated into a global market and have access to the global governance complex, to which the UN belongs. In contrast, vast amounts of people—women, gays, lesbians, transvestites, transgender people remain excluded. They are clearly much more vulnerable to gender hatred and sex wars. A major challenge is, then, to connect issues of sexual differences to social and economic dimensions, to think of sexual rights as social and economic rights in order to bring people together around common causes.

44 Global impact

US sexual health and reproductive policy

Renée T. White and Cynthia Pope

Rose Wanjera was one of the lucky ones. A Kenyan widow in her mid-twenties, Wanjera was suffering from pregnancy related complications, according to a 2003 *New York Times* article. She went to a local clinic funded by Marie Stopes International (MSI). There, she received help and immediately enrolled in a maternal healthcare program.

Had Wanjera's problems happened today, she might not have received the care she needed. MSI, known internationally for their healthcare for the poor, has recently lost all of its funding from the United States Agency for International Development (USAID). As a result, MSI Kenya had to close two of their twenty-one clinics, lay off more than eighty medical professionals, and reduce comprehensive care services offered in the remaining clinics.

MSI lost USAID funding due to a June 2002 reactivation of the Mexico City Plan, also known as the Global Gag Rule. The Global Gag Rule no longer allows distribution of USAID funds to nongovernmental organizations (NGOs) that either provide or discuss abortion, or if they advocate less restrictive abortion laws in their own countries. MSI refused to sign the Global Gag Rule.

The challenges of the Global Gag Rule that confront MSI are also faced by other well-established family planning and comprehensive health NGOs such as the London-based International Planned Parenthood Association (PPA). In Zambia, PPA has lost 24 percent of its USAID funding and is no longer allowed to share contraceptive supplies with smaller NGOs. Lesotho, where 25 percent of women live with HIV/AIDS, is one of twenty-nine developing countries no longer receiving any USAID-supplied condoms. In Ethiopia, Amare Badada, of the Ethiopian Family Guidance Association, refused to sign the gag rule as well. According to a 2003 BBC article, since then, one region—Nazareth—had to close forty-four of their fifty-four clinics. "Under the gag rule, I can treat a woman who comes bleeding after an illegal abortion but I am not allowed to warn her of the dangers before she goes." One of the MSI clinics that is now closed—Mathare Valley clinic in Nairobi—was the only healthcare resource for approximately 300,000 people.

In each of these situations, US policies have direct and measurable impacts on the global provision of family planning and family health services—services can make the difference between life and death. The World Health Organization estimates that every minute 380 women become pregnant, 190 women face an unplanned or unwanted pregnancy, 110 women experience a pregnancy-related complication, 40 women have an unsafe abortion, and one woman dies. A review of policies from the 1960s through current times shows that as the domestic political pendulum swings on sexual and reproductive rights, so too do US policies on global reproductive health.

Foreign aid for family planning

The 1960s marked a period of innovative policy and program development in the United States. The United States first allocated foreign assistance for family planning with the Foreign Assistance Act of 1961, which provided funds for research on family planning and the provision of family planning resources. By the 1970s the United States became the major contributor to the United Nations Fund for Population Activities (UNFPA). This fund was to serve three main purposes: to reduce poverty, raise standards of living, and improve health. The US administration recognized that these three goals were the central tenets of a human rights framework.

Support for generous international and domestic family planning funding continued through the 1970s, but a shift in the national reproductive rights debate began to be felt internationally. In 1973, the year that abortion was legalized in the United States, Congress passed the Helms Amendment to the Foreign Assistance Act (FAA). The Helms Amendment prohibited the direct use of US foreign assistance for abortion services in nations receiving FAA funding. Thus, by the time Ronald Reagan was elected president in 1980, reproductive health and family planning had been redefined as "abortion services" and public discussion of reproductive health was increasingly cast in moral terms. Since the Reagan administration a series of initiatives have attempted to reinforce the association between family planning, reproductive rights, and abortion.

Presidents Reagan and George H.W. Bush represented a sea change in how the United States carries out its role in global reproductive health policy. They broke from previous international policies and human rights-centered approaches. One of the targets was abortion. The Reagan administration did not get domestic support for its anti-abortion stance, so it looked to the international arena to put laws in place.

As such, in 1984 Reagan enforced the Global Gag Rule, also known as the Mexico City Policy, which put his abortion rhetoric to action; the Reagan administration would no longer disburse USAID funding to NGOs that either provided or discussed abortion. In 1985 the Kemp Kasten Amendment, which was attached to the Foreign Operations Appropriations Act, stipulated that no federal money would go toward "coercive abortion or involuntary sterilization." This was a reaction to China's one-child policy. The US president was the person to determine to which cases this rule applied. When considered together, the Global Gag Rule and the Kemp Kasten Amendment function as anti-abortion policies, not as ones intended to further women's health or human rights abroad.

President Clinton rescinded this Global Gag Rule soon after he assumed office. The Clinton administration assumed a leadership role in the 1994 Cairo International Conference on Population and Development (ICPD) and was one of the key actors that drafted the Programme of Action. One of the important conference results was the signing of the 2015 Goal: to provide reproductive and sexual health services for all citizens in the world, thus reducing maternal mortality and HIV prevalence rates.

After the Clinton administration's eight-year international commitment to reproductive and human rights, the United States is experiencing a return to a pre-Clinton ideology. In July 2002 Bush repealed $34 million in committed funds to UNFPA (As Francoise Girard notes in *Global Implications of Domestic and International Policies on Sexuality* [2004], 12 percent of the fund's annual budget) because it operates in China, which since the 1970s has had a one child per family policy. The State Department said the money would be redirected to family planning programs in thirteen

African countries, but it was eventually used for unrelated projects in Afghanistan and Pakistan.

Ironically, more abortions are likely to result from the current cuts in reproductive health funds. In the executive summary of *Access Denied: US Restrictions on International Family Planning*, the authors observe that:

> When the [Mexico City] policy was previously in effect, however, from 1984 to 1992, there was little evidence that the policy reduced the incidence of abortion, as women continued to seek clandestine procedures. There is little reason to believe it will be any more effective this time around. In practice, the policy is likely to have the opposite effect; it will reduce access to contraception, leading to more unwanted and high-risk pregnancies, more unsafe abortions, and more maternal illness, injury, and even death.

Family health clinics around the world have been forced to cut services, and many clinics have been shut down, thus denying citizens access to any sort of medical care, increasing the "global burden of disease." According to a 2004 "Issues in Brief" circulated by the Guttmacher Institute, this global burden of disease can be calculated as an annual loss of 250 million years of production due to death or disability resulting from poor sexual and reproductive health.

A question of human rights

In response to the tenth anniversary of the United State's commitment to the ICPD, the current administration has verbally renewed support for the Programme of Action. However, actions speak louder then words. The Global Gag Rule is still in place and the $15 billion President's Emergency Plan for AIDS Relief (PEPFAR) is beginning to have global impacts. For example, in *The War on Choice*, Gloria Feldt, president of Planned Parenthood Federation of America reports that:

> Already there are 78,000 deaths from unsafe abortions each year, and the continued enforcement of the gag rule will only make that number go up. Deaths by AIDS have increased measurably . . . Under the gag rule, some countries have been unable to maintain their level of contraceptive supplies and healthcare services, many clinics have closed, and family planning providers are having more difficulty working with the governments to coordinate healthcare.

The Global Gag Rule, since reactivation, has resulted in the closing of clinics in Bangladesh, Ghana, and Kenya. These anti-abortion policies also play into the PEPFAR policies. Suzanne Goldberg reports in an October 2004 *Observer* article that the spill-over effect from the Global Gag Rule casts an ideological shadow on PEPFAR. Instead of relying on experienced organizations and the Global Fund for AIDS, the first phase of the funding has been channeled through faith-based organizations that support an abstinence-only, no-condom agenda to halting the spread of HIV.

In Ethiopia, for example, the Orthodox Church was awarded $5 million to work on HIV prevention. In Nigeria as well, the bulk of the $5 million in aid will be distributed through primarily Christian faith-based organizations.

In 2006 the administration implemented a requirement that at least one-third of all HIV-prevention funds be devoted to abstinence-only programs. Ironically, Bush has heralded Uganda's dramatic reduction in rates of HIV transmission. However, this reduction was not due to abstinence but rather due to the availability of condoms and the promotion of monogamy. "People are frustrated," says Adrienne Germain, president of the International Women's Health Coalition. "The legislators who are in control right now firmly believe that everyone can and should simply abstain until marriage and have only one partner in marriage ever in life, and that is totally contrary to reality."

Given the tenth-year anniversary and the continuation of PEPFAR global funding, it is imperative to revisit the issue of reproductive and sexual health in terms of human rights. Since 1965 US organizations have generally been recognized as leaders in the family planning field, so one must ask whether US global health policy will shape how other nations prioritize their international health aid.

45 Abstinence goes global

The United States, the right wing, and human rights

Cynthia Rothschild

A range of organizations has pointed out that the Bush administration has made vital public health decisions based, not on scientifically proven fact, but on ideology. Since this article first appeared in 2003, the Bush administration has continued to promote, and filter resources to, abstinence and abstinence-only-until-marriage programs. Whether through HIV prevention or anti-violence programs, funds have been directed to discriminatory, anti-sex and ideologically driven efforts with significant human rights and public health implications, many of which have direct impact on women. Of particular concern is the President's Emergency Plan for AIDS Relief (PEPFAR), which continues to channel a significant proportion of global HIV prevention funds to abstinence-only programs. From AIDS organizations to the American Civil Liberties Union (ACLU), groups in the United States have argued that abstinence-only programs constitute a lethal form of censorship by withholding information on methods known to prevent HIV and STI (sexually transmitted infection) transmission.

Since its earliest days the administration has promoted abstinence-only-until-marriage programs as its preferred means of HIV prevention. A like-minded Congress approved over $120 million for domestic abstinence programs in its fiscal year 2003 budget, $50 million of which was connected to the US Welfare Reform Act and to programs that teach that a "mutually faithful monogamous relationship in the context of marriage is the expected standard of human sexual activity." These federally funded initiatives limit all discussion of contraceptives—and condoms—to a focus on their failure rates.

Most organizations concentrate on US domestic concerns about abstinence-only education and funding. However, it is also vital to consider the global arena, where the US administration exports its sectarian ideology and morality, primarily through restrictions on foreign assistance funds and the policy positions of US delegations at the United Nations. Both domestically and internationally, scientifically sound arguments could be strengthened by use of a human rights perspective, namely one that rests on the ideas enshrined in the Universal Declaration of Human Rights and other internationally agreed instruments that *all people have the right to information, to education, to enjoy the benefits of scientific progress, to be free from discrimination, to freedom of expression and to enjoy the highest attainable standard of health*. Taken together, these and other standards form the basis of international human rights law. The denial of these rights, and others, in relation to public health threatens each person's right to life and constitutes an infringement of international law for which governments, including the current US administration, must be held accountable.

Human rights organizations are especially well positioned to address abstinence-only programs as a rights issue. In doing so they could hold governments accountable for human rights violations inherent in the implementation of many abstinence-only programs, which are enforced through discriminatory and moralistic restrictions on what can and cannot be taught or discussed. They could build coalitions between domestic and international groups concerned with public health and discrimination. They could also capitalize on the opportunity to develop their own advocacy positions on gender and health.

The people who have the most to gain from collaborative work grounded in human rights analysis are those who need and want information but are denied accurate, scientifically proven information about disease prevention and transmission, condom use, and contraception. While false and misleading information about health jeopardizes the well-being of all people, certain groups are at particular risk when accurate information is censored, altered, or withheld. These include women and young people (particularly girls) and people who are already marginalized, including sex workers, lesbian, gay, bisexual and transgender people, and people who inject drugs.

US abstinence agenda: policy without proof

Fictional claims, manipulation of information, and imposition of gag rules are emerging as three consistent tools in the administration's implementation of its domestic and international public health agenda. This is especially true where sexuality and reproductive rights are concerned. The Bush administration's First Secretary of Health and Human Services, who was also the chair of the Global Fund to Fight AIDS, Tuberculosis and Malaria, justified increased domestic spending on abstinence-only programs knowing that there was no credible proof that they were effective. At the time, these posts were held by Tommy G. Thompson who once said: "Let's try them out and see if we can't get it to work." The policy, in effect, denies scientifically proven methods of reducing HIV transmission in order to promote an idea that is popular with a core of conservative Republican voters.

In this administration, the desire to "make abstinence work" trumps the human right to life. The consequences of these skewed priorities are deadly, especially as young people constitute one of the groups with the most rapidly rising rates of HIV infection. US polices are, in effect, eliminating one of the only tools available that can save people's lives: information.

In Congress, right-wing policy makers such as Rep. Chris Smith (R-NJ) and Rep. Joseph Pitts (R-PA) have worked to ensure that programs with no medically proven effectiveness have been funded. Political pressure also has been used to de-fund family planning programs (such as the United Nations Family Planning Association). HIV prevention and other sexuality education programs have been audited when their work was seen to stray from the abstinence-only line. While there is a growing list of organizations that have been targeted, two examples are worth noting: San Francisco's Stop AIDS program faced over a year of continuous federal reviews, and Advocates for Youth endured three audits in one year.

One of the more egregious examples of Congressional efforts to promote abstinence-only ideology in the international arena is directly pegged to fighting the AIDS pandemic. Even though the US administration called for $15 billion to fight AIDS in Africa and the Caribbean, the Congressional budget appropriations process shows this commitment to be subject to conservative ideological constraints. Congress earmarked one-third of prevention funds to programs that promote abstinence-only ideology, and reduced funding for comprehensive prevention efforts that have shown positive results.

Members of Congress and the administration, in part, justify this allocation of funds by touting the success of abstinence programs in Uganda, even though public health officials in Uganda and elsewhere question the validity of those claims. *The Lancet* medical journal reported on July 6, 2002 that increased condom use also contributed to the decline in prevalence rates and that conclusions crediting only the abstinence portion of Uganda's AIDS-prevention programs are based on scientifically unsound data collection and manipulation of numbers.

Policies from Washington are fundamentally flawed because they ignore the realities of millions of people, particularly women and girls, all over the globe. Abstinence is meaningless for many women and girls who have limited or no power to negotiate condom use or to resist violence by male partners or strangers. There are 82 million young women in developing countries currently between the ages of ten and seventeen who will marry before their eighteenth birthdays. It is foolish to insist that these young women "just say no" to sex demanded by their older and more powerful husbands. In many scenarios it is the husbands who have the power to abstain; too often, they don't and their young wives can't.

The United States and abstinence at the United Nations

Many of the same groups that promote the most conservative and restrictive policies on sexual and reproductive rights domestically are appearing on the global scene, and in recent UN meetings related to health, children, and population issues. In these settings US delegations have attempted to insert abstinence in their negotiations on international agreements and have protested if abstinence provisions were removed. In many of these meetings, the US administration worked directly with advisers from right-wing organizations such as the Family Research Council (FRC), Focus on the Family (FoF), and Concerned Women for America (CWA). Whether in relation to abstinence specifically, or reproductive rights more generally, US delegation statements and positions reflect a swing to an extremist ideology.

At the UN General Assembly Special Session on Children in 2002, the US delegation, which included FRC and CWA, tried to block international consensus on comprehensive sexuality education and related services for young people. In an official written explanation of its position, the delegation emphasized its "commitment to programs that address . . . the need to stress the practices of abstinence, of delaying sexual initiation, monogamy, fidelity and partner reduction" to prevent HIV infection. In its positions, the US delegation supported myopic and moralistic domestic policies that sought to position abstinence as the only worthwhile method of reducing transmission.

In 2002, over thirty Asian countries voted against conservative US positions at an important regional meeting on population and development in Bangkok. At the end of the meeting, the entirely isolated US delegation issued an official statement on the final agreed document. The statement repeats the language from the earlier meeting on children and adds that the "United States made every effort to insert language in the document reaffirming the importance of abstinence" and "remains disappointed" that the assertion that "abstinence is the healthiest choice for unmarried adolescents" was deleted from the final text.

During 2004 and 2005, in regional and global meetings related to the tenth anniversaries of the International Conference on Population and Development ("the Cairo conference") and the Fourth World Conference on Women ("the Beijing conference"), US delegations persistently advocated for inclusion of references to abstinence in documents under negotiation by governments. At many of these meetings, the US delegations issued official "statements of explanation," which elaborated on the US government's commitment to abstinence and on the limitations of their interpretations of references to abortion.

Resistance

Disinformation and ideologically driven funding are beginning to be challenged. Feminist and reproductive rights organizations, such as Catholics for a Free Choice, the Center for Health and Gender Equity, Development Alternatives with Women for a New Era, and the International Women's Health Coalition, are working to counter extremist ideologues at the United Nations and in other global policy fora. Progressive coalitions of nongovernmental organizations are cooperating with ally delegations here and overseas to share accurate information about comprehensive sexuality education and to strengthen the ability to refute abstinence-only messages.

There is clear progress domestically as well. Human Rights Watch compiled a bold and first-of-its-kind report critiquing abstinence-only programs in Texas. Rep. Henry Waxman (D-CA) recently issued a report criticizing the Bush administration's persistent misuse and manipulation of science. Whistleblowers persist within the National Institute of Health and the Centers for Disease Control, despite being pressured to alter or suppress scientifically accurate information. And AIDS service organizations have begun to decry the prioritization of abstinence in US global AIDS funding.

The right wing has been very effective at melding its domestic and global strategies. Progressive organizations and social movements must do the same, and with urgency. Using a human rights lens to critique abstinence-only programs and the manipulation of valid scientific data would go a long way in fostering effective coalitions. Coalitions of human rights organizations, and sexual and reproductive health and rights organizations, must increasingly take their fight to global and UN levels to protect gains already won.

Organizations working in domestic and international arenas would do well to build on one another's analyses and work together to challenge the current administration's "make abstinence work" philosophy and to expose its strong links with conservative extremist advisors. We must do this by deploying a variety of rights-based arguments and by making a renewed and passionate commitment to linking the domestic with the global.

46 Sex work in contemporary Vietnam

Foreign plague or homegrown problem?

Christophe Robert

Teenage Vietnamese girls in high heels and short skirts crowd around sunburned, sweating, middle-aged white men in a bar in central Saigon. It's hot and dark outside; inside, the music is loud, the beer cold. Young women smile and giggle, teasing the men in broken English. They stand in the doorways of bars and hail the foreign tourists who pass by in the street.

The scene is familiar, too much so, perhaps. This type of Asian prostitution is immediately recognizable. It forms part of the common stock of images inherited from Hollywood films and from the Vietnam War, and is reminiscent of representations and practices of prostitution in other cities in Southeast Asia, from Thailand to the Philippines. And yet this image may say more about the fantasies of Western journalists than about the realities of prostitution since the "open door" period of the 1990s, when the Vietnamese Communist Party instituted market-oriented reforms. Anthropological research, such as the project I conducted in Ho Chi Minh City (still commonly referred to as Saigon)—which includes interviews and discussions with prostitutes, journalists, civil servants, and members of various nongovernmental organizations involved in HIV/AIDS prevention and care—can provide a more realistic picture of prostitution and social problems in Vietnam.

Statistics on the extent of prostitution in Vietnam are unreliable, varying from around 60,000 to over 200,000 female prostitutes. Police and security agencies favor the latter, unrealistically high estimates, in order to support their repressive approaches to the problem. State agencies and organizations use unreliable and often fraudulent data in the war of words and turf battles to assert control over prostitution. In addition, Vietnamese state-controlled media have promoted the image of prostitutes catering primarily to foreign men in an attempt to account for the imagined perils of the market economy, with HIV/AIDS as the new foreign-born plague. In the 1990s newspapers started featuring moralizing stories about greedy young female prostitutes in new foreign-tourist neighborhoods, with titillating titles such as "'Sentimental Services' in the Western Backpacker District" (*Phu Nu* [Woman], Sunday edition, November 6, 2005, p. 6). Photographs are an important aspect of these stories. They show young women dressed provocatively and made up in ways that seem foreign to the majority of Vietnamese who have no access to these new tourist neighborhoods. The official response of the government is ideological but vague, as evidenced from Directive 14-CT (1993), which states, "In our country today, prostitution is growing, with negative consequences for the cultural life of our society, for social order and peace among our people, and polluting the moral traditions and beautiful customs of our nation." Similarly, government decrees 05/CP, 87/CP, and 88/CP (1996) state that prostitution combines three kinds of danger: a threat to public health, a source of crime and disorder, and cultural pollution and moral degeneration.

This representation hides important parts of the puzzle of social problems in Vietnam in the 1990s. The very visible sex trade with white foreigners masks the existence of much less visible, but more prevalent, local forms of prostitution between Vietnamese, as well as cases of HIV/AIDS transmission that have nothing to do with foreigners. Linking prostitution to the arrival of foreign male tourists, thirsty for alcohol and hungry for drugs and sex, takes the focus off the domestic sex trade sector in Vietnam under socialism.

It is true that establishments catering to a foreign male clientele—with English-only names such as Apocalypse Now, Gossip, Hazard—sprang up in Vietnamese cities in the 1990s. They are a reminder of "R&R" ("rest and relaxation") during the Vietnam War when American soldiers heavily patronized Vietnamese prostitutes. But, now as then, these establishments open and remain open only thanks to formal authorizations and informal arrangements, such as bribes and favors to the local police. When pressed by journalists, government officials answer that the situation is "complex," and promise better coordination between various police agencies. An interview with Nguyen Ngoc Thach, Head of the Ho Chi Minh City Office of the Campaign against Social Evils in *Phu Nu* (Woman) magazine (November 6, 2005) exemplifies this position. The Vietnamese media criticizes these establishments for their sleaziness, and rightly so. They also criticize young female prostitutes for their greed and laziness, and for violating ideals of the soft-spoken, obedient, hardworking Vietnamese woman. For example, a typical headline from the hugely popular tabloid newspaper *Public Security* (published by the Public Security of Ho Chi Minh City) reads, "Committing crimes stems from an unwholesome life" (May 18, 2000, p. 26). The article blames prostitutes and drug addicts for fostering criminality.

This type of criticism assigns blame for social problems on scapegoat groups, as opposed to treating prostitution or drug use as symptoms of larger social dysfunctions, such as poverty. We can set up the problem differently and note that the development of the market economy in Vietnam in the 1990s has created tremendous opportunities, while fostering economic inequalities. Aren't young female prostitutes, then, showing entrepreneurial spirit? Are they not being dutiful daughters, bowing down to the oft-asserted ideal of filial piety and feminine obedience? Aren't young women from the countryside being recruited to work as karaoke hostesses or waitresses, while their families know that their real occupation is prostitution and benefit from the remittances the daughters send home every month?

Male urges and women's work

Foreign tourism did not single handedly give rise to prostitution in Vietnam today. A commercial sex sector catering to foreign tourists does exist. Yet explaining prostitution this way obscures broader gender issues and socioeconomic problems.

A new class of wealthy Vietnamese businessmen emerged in the 1990s. Thanks to their connections with government officials, these men received large contracts in the transition from a state-run to a more liberalized economy. They display their status and wealth by gathering in expensive restaurants and karaoke bars and by patronizing prostitutes. The common practice of inviting one's clients or bosses to clinch a deal or curry favor usually includes a meeting with hostesses who also provide sexual services. At the other end of the economic scale, a lot of poor, uneducated, younger men have not reaped the benefits of economic development. In interviews they say that they are now too poor to be attractive marriage partners so they turn to prostitutes to relieve "sexual urges." In Vietnam, these male urges are assumed to be irresistible and to require discharge; common wisdom, then, reinforces the normalization of prostitution. Men from various socioeconomic classes use the commodified bodies of prostitutes to relieve their sexual urges. Female prostitutes stroke male egos, buttress insecure masculinities, and act as status symbols for the wealthy and powerful.

Shifting focus away from foreign men as the cause of social problems brings to light Vietnamese cultural patterns that may be intertwined with sex work. Sex work in Vietnam is far from new and far from radically threatening the social order, contrary to what media representations and government officials assert. Perhaps, then, sex work is a continuation, now in the market economy, of long-standing forms of female work in the family.

Notions of womanhood in Vietnam idealize a female who has little self-interest: a woman finds true realization of who she is only through marriage and through giving birth to children, preferably sons who will continue the family line. Her fulfillment, economically, socially, and sexually, is not the question. The question instead is to insure that through a web of obligations and demands on her body and mind she submits willingly to these demands. This is the primary goal of education in the family and in state institutions, which often rely on strategically redefined Confucian values. Yet, if we study the history of Vietnam, we see that far from being a cultural bedrock of Vietnamese society, "Confucianism," with its emphasis on hierarchy and duty, has been used to assert conservative and repressive agendas and stifle social dissent, particularly from subjugated groups, such as the rural poor, women, and youth. Anthropology, the practice of encounters and interviews with actual people, enables us to question current assertions of conservative leaders that "Confucian values" or even "traditional Vietnamese culture" ought to dictate the proper behavior of women.

By publicizing the question of prostitution the Vietnamese media highlight the contradictions in women's roles in society. The image of deviant young women cavorting with foreign, white men is convenient. It helps avoid the more complicated questions of who benefits from the sex work of these young women and from the work of women throughout Vietnamese society.

In interviews Vietnamese women complain that their contributions to family life are not recognized, since their husbands or their families take them for granted. They are expected to perform domestic chores and to contribute to the household budget by working outside the home. And yet, women say, most men bristle when they are asked to share some of the domestic chores. Women complain that their husbands routinely patronize prostitutes. Notions that this is "what men do" contribute further to the normalization of prostitution. In this context, why assume that prostitution strictly results from the evils of contact with foreigners and the market economy?

Following what Vietnamese women themselves say, a better way to pose the question would be to argue that the prevalence of commercial sex work stems from tensions in gender roles in Vietnam today. A good place to start would be to examine Vietnamese women's daily lives and note how notions of marriage, sexuality, child rearing, education, even the very notion of the family are changing much more rapidly than political or media discourses about them. This shift helps explain why the official demonization of female prostitutes is so popular in Vietnam today: leaders are trying to reassert some sense of control over social realities that escape their grasp, in particular over the beginnings of the emancipation of women who are becoming educated and joining the workforce in ever larger numbers.

47 The moral economy of sex in Russia

Jakob Rigi

In the global market for sex, some of the most valuable women are from Russia.

As with other post-Socialist countries, when the Soviet Union collapsed, sex became a commodity and thousands if not millions of women—and men—were eager to trade. Several dynamics led to this growth. Reforms that replaced communism with capitalism, coupled with a scarcity of well-paying jobs, forced many women to get involved in sex work in order to survive. The dismantling of the welfare state undermined the service sector (mostly healthcare and education), which was the primary employer of women. These traditionally female jobs were devalued and salaries for them decreased. Many women lost their jobs all together.

At the same time, these neo-liberal reforms created a small class of wealthy capitalists. For many women, the only access to an expanding consumerist culture was through rich men, either through kinship or through sexual relationship. If not the daughter of a capitalist, women were the wives, lovers, or prostitutes of these men. Advertisements and pornography propagated new idealized images of sexy female bodies and people began questioning the former sexual morality, which focused on women as mothers and workers. This was the beginning of a radical and commercialized sexual revolution in the former Soviet bloc. The consumption of women's bodies as sexualized commodities became part of capitalist's masculine and social identities.

Still, Russians have very diverse moral attitudes toward sex work. Rural populations and the older generation tend to find sex work or prostitution reprehensible. Prior to the Soviet Era women's identity in official discourses was based on their contribution as mothers to the family and as workers to society. Although prostitution existed marginally, the sale of women's bodies was considered wrong. Men's identity was determined mostly through their social position and the ways their work was useful to society as a whole. In the family men were considered the primary breadwinners.

The younger generation, though, tends not to pass moral judgment on sex work. The following discussion, which took place in St Petersburg in the summer of 2003 with three Ph.D. students, illustrates this attitude. These young people were blasé about sex work and found nothing wrong with prostitution, reflecting their embrace of neo-liberal ideology. In this ideology everything is for sale, including the body and soul. The conversation was drawn from a larger anthropological research project, which considers the radical changes related to sexuality that occurred in Russia since the end of the Soviet era.

VLADIMIR: Our society with regard to sexuality is a very cunning society. It is erotic but also hierarchical. No one in this city can live without money. Telephone, gas, electricity, and all other goods and services—without money these are not available. If there is money you can keep the city going on. In the sexual sphere it is the same: without money you cannot do anything. Even people who think their relations are not based on money rely on money for their relations.

JAKOB: Sex is the exchange of two bodies. Why must one pay for it?

IRENA: Well if I have sex with someone, it means that I am giving something, and so I must get something in exchange. In this way it is a kind of exchange. In exchange equivalents are exchanged. If I give you sex, you must give me money. Anyway, in order to have good sex, you need to have good material conditions.

VLADIMIR: You cannot do it on the street; you need to do it at home.

IRENA: You need a good apartment and clean sheets.

JULIA: For me to be able to do it, I need to drink good wine and eat good food.

JAKOB: But this is not exactly what I mean by commoditization of sexuality.

VLADIMIR: Well the obvious form is when people hire prostitutes. But there are other forms. Say a woman goes to a shop and there she meets a man who invites her to a good restaurant. There, he buys her good wine and good food and gets her expensive presents. She will be very happy that someone has paid so much attention to her. And she may sleep with him.

JAKOB: But other people have told me that this is a Russian tradition, for a man to "wine and dine" a woman and then expect sex in exchange.

VLADIMIR: People buy sex for themselves but then call it the Russian tradition. Others are more honest; they go to sex shops and buy pornography, rather than buying women. But both buy sex. Prostitution is a financial operation.

IRENA: There is nothing horrible about it. If you need bread, you go to the shop and buy it. If you need sex, you go to the street and buy it.

JAKOB: I think that there is a difference between sex that is non-commercial and the buying of a woman's body as a commodity. In sex, both partners are actively engaged. In prostitution one side is active, while the prostitute is reduced to an object, not unlike the example you give of bread . . .

JULIA: That is bullshit. You have it completely wrong. What is an object and what is objectification? If I am on the street and working [as a prostitute] a man will ask me to go home with him and I will. He will behave like a gentleman. He will gently touch my breasts, he will caress me, and he will tell me, "If you don't want to go home with me, we can meet each other another time and befriend each other, and then we will do it."

JAKOB: But maybe what you are talking about is an exception. I interviewed prostitutes in Kazakhstan. They told me that for them there was essentially no difference between their clients and the condoms they used—that is they were both just objects that were part of the business, not really human beings. The only difference is that the clients paid money.

IRENA: We are talking about different types of prostitutes. When I go to the street I am ready to sell my body, but I can sell it in different ways. If I don't like the client, then I am an object. If I like him, then I am not. I can have emotions and pleasure.

JULIA: As long as there is emotion, there is no objectification. I have a friend who is a prostitute. She speaks with clients and chooses those she likes and rejects the others. She enjoys having sex with them but may receive money as well. You can work as a librarian in different ways; you can also fuck men in different ways.

VLADIMIR: Our prostitutes are different. Sometimes they don't take money from men they like. I have a friend who was a pimp in a brothel in Germany, and he told me that they had difficulty in convincing some Russian girls to take money from their favorite clients. Here our prostitutes may not charge a client whom they like. In Germany this is not possible because the pimps will not allow it. Marriage is like prostitution. A man and a woman marry and the husband supports the wife; it is a contract.

JAKOB: Will you practice prostitution?

IRENA: Of course I would if it were safe. Yes, if I had a good figure, and if I had a good pimp who could protect me. Some men are maniacs.

JULIA: You have a strange image of prostitution. I don't want to sleep with a man who has no money. Nobody will marry someone who doesn't have a car and a good salary and cannot provide her with a good material life. What is the difference? Prostitution is cheaper.

JAKOB: How do people relate morally to prostitution?

IRENA: They think it is okay.

VLADIMIR: The prostitutes are spiritual.

JAKOB: What is the social morality on this?

IRENA: There is not a common morality; people have different opinions.

VLADIMIR: Some people may publicly denounce prostitution, but in private they are jealous of prostitutes. Many women who cannot engage in prostitution dream of doing so.

IRENA: If her occupation is formally prostitution, people do not condemn it.

VLADIMIR: But if she does it hypocritically, people may condemn it.

JAKOB: If you were to fall in love with a girl who is a prostitute, would you marry her?

VLADIMIR : Yes, but I will try to convince her to change her job.

JAKOB: Why? If I love an accountant I will not ask her to change her job.

VLADIMIR: It would be difficult with sexual relations.

JAKOB: Why? Do you mean morally?

VLADIMIR: Not morally but practically. There is no morality here. My previous wife was a prostitute.

JAKOB: Are you kidding?

VLADIMIR: Of course not. It is better. If a prostitute chooses you as her husband, it means that you are the greatest man because she has experienced so many different men.

JAKOB: You said something about *soderzhanka* [a woman who is a lover of a well off man and gets financial support from him; or a "kept woman"].

IRENA: Well any woman is soderzhanka. A woman who does not get money is ready to go to a good niche (*Khorshia Nisha*) in order to earn money. It is really a good thing. A prostitute is in a much better situation than a soderzhanka. A soderzhanka is living like a slave, waiting for the man and always looking to his hands for money, while the prostitute has her own money and decides about her own life and time. Soderzhanka is materially and emotionally dependent on her sponsor, insecure. She suffers a lot while the prostitute does not suffer. She does not wait for the man to appear at the door, to be available at his will and always at his service.

JAKOB: Why, then, are older people against prostitution?

IRENA: These old people are the children of *Komsomol* [the communist party's youth organization in the USSR] and their supposedly Orthodox attitudes come from

Komsomol, not from the Orthodox Church. Anti-prostitution morality really comes from the Soviet era.

The attitudes reflected by Vladimir, Julia, and Irena about sex work in Russia are widespread among youth in St Petersburg. For them, sex work is similar to any other kind of work and, for many in the younger generation, it should be recognized as such rather than stigmatized. However, we also find that other perspectives, from the older generation as well as young people, consider prostitution an immoral practice and they patently condemn it. The growth of prostitution, coupled with these contradictory moral values about it are symptoms of wide-reaching changes in Russia that can be called "post-Soviet capitalism." In this form of capitalism, many aspects of life such as education, knowledge, and sexuality, which were previously outside the purview of a market economy, have been transformed into commodities that can be bought and sold.

48 Nicaragua's changing erotiscapes

Hot bed of cold war takes on sexual rights

Cymene Howe

In the swelter of a June afternoon, Carlos* and I sat together drinking sweet coffee in front of his sister's pink house in a working-class neighborhood in Managua, Nicaragua's capital. As part of my anthropological research on sexual and gender rights in contemporary Nicaragua, Carlos and I were meeting to discuss his early days of activism for sexual rights in Nicaragua in the 1980s. He explained:

> We went to the media, we went to the radio and the TV and we sat down and we said, "we are homosexuals, we are lesbians and we want you to respect our rights. That you respect our human rights. We are all equal to whoever. We are good kids, we are good fathers, we are good mothers, we are good neighbors and we are good workers. Equal. There are bad ones too, like everyone. But we are humans and here we are."

Carlos's comment may seem common enough from the perspective of lesbian and gay rights movements in the United States, but in Nicaragua the remark is striking. When Carlos began his activist work, the revolutionary regime of the Sandinistas held power and while the socialist-inspired agenda of the Sandinistas made wide reaching changes in Nicaragua's distribution of wealth, including increasing education and health services for the impoverished masses, the government's reforms focused on the liberation of "the people" as whole. That often meant sidestepping the specific concerns of sexual minorities and women. The Sandinistas did not practice the heavy-handed persecution of homosexual men and women as had been the case in Cuba, but neither were sexual rights part of the Sandinistas' social agenda.

Currently, Nicaragua is the second poorest country in the Western Hemisphere. In a place where whole sectors of the population are victims of what international development experts call "extreme poverty," social activism takes on a degree of urgency. By necessity, scarce human and material resources must be channeled into effective campaigns and there is a delicate balance that must be struck between economic, social, and human rights. Sexual rights advocacy in Nicaragua must have broad transformative potential, as activists aim to reconfigure cultural meanings regarding sexual values and behaviors. But Nicaragua, partly because of its revolutionary experience, is a place quite familiar with social change.

Since the end of the revolutionary era in 1990, the Nicaraguan government has made the country's anti-sodomy law (Article 204) more virulent with increased prison

*Names changed to protect privacy.

sentences. International human rights organizations have dubbed the law "the most repressive in all of Latin America." Article 204 indicts not only men who practice homosexual acts, but women as well, making it unusual among anti-sodomy legislation around the world. While the law is not widely enforced, it threatens not only those who participate in same sex sexual behavior, but also those who "promote or propagandize homosexuality"—a category that could include newspaper reporters, therapists, and activists. Sexual and gender rights advocates and nongovernmental organizations (NGOs) around the country have protested the regressive legislation, asserting its unconstitutionality and receiving broad support from international advocacy organizations.

Despite Article 204, an annual "sexuality free from prejudice" (*una sexualidad libre de prejuicios*) celebration is held every June in cities around Nicaragua. The events include film screenings (such as *Fresa y Chocolate*, *Boys Don't Cry*, *Ma Vie en Rose*), research presentations, talks by experts in the field of sexuality, discussion groups, radio programs and not surprisingly, a great final party. During the rest of the year transvestic beauty pageants are regular fare at the *discos gay* in Managua, and local NGOs host rap groups about lesbian and gay identity and HIV prevention. These are some of the ways in which gender and sexuality activists, working together on what they see as related vectors of inequality, are attempting to craft interventions for social justice in what many described as a "very socially conservative" and "hostile" environment. Community members and organizations are attempting to change an ethos in Nicaragua that makes lesbians largely invisible, places *hombres efeminados* (effeminate men) at the center of derision, and in the most extreme cases, mandates up to four years in prison.

What does it mean to be *"lesbiana"* or *"gay"*, *"cochóna"* or *"cochón"* in Nicaragua?

In the past, Nicaraguans, like many in Latin America, have not rigidly separated male homosexuality from male heterosexuality; neither did they designate a "sexual identity" based on homoerotic behavior. Rather, cultural assumptions have focused on men's role—as either a "passive" or "active" partner in the sex act. In other words, it is not *whether* a man had sex with another man, but *how*. Men were stigmatized as a *cochón* (loosely translated as "fag") based upon the presumed role played in homoerotic encounters. In the past *cochones* never accrued the respect that the putatively "real men" who had insertive sex with them did, and they were the target of *burla*, or mockery—often because of their failure to conform to gender roles.

Unfortunately, women's same sex sexuality has been largely ignored in studies of sexuality in Nicaragua, leaving the question of how women conceive of their same sex relationships and desires largely unanswered. What is clear, however, is that women who are considered "too masculine" (*"marimacha"* or *"cochóna"* [dyke]) face much more stigma than do feminine appearing women who may also have affective and sexual relationships with other women.

Now in Nicaragua a new era appears to be in the making. The categories of *"homosexual,"* *"gay,"* and *"lesbiana"* are becoming more pervasive particularly in Nicaragua's urban centers. Consequently, many men and women are identifying with, while at the same time being stigmatized by, these terms. These discursive changes and the emergence of sexual identities in Nicaragua mirror transformations globally, as cities in most countries can now claim organizations or social movements that advocate for lesbian and gay rights. Concepts about sexual rights and a kind of universally recognizable homosexual subject now circulate on the world stage.

However, as identity politics in the United States have demonstrated, there are many ways in which identities operate: sometimes to the benefit of self-constituted minority groups and sometimes to the detriment of those who are accused of asserting "special privileges" or rights. The case is likewise complex in Nicaragua. Adding to this complexity is the question of whether categories such as "lesbian" and "gay" are well suited to the Nicaraguan context; these identity monikers have been, at various times, criticized as "foreign imports" from Europe and the United States. Given Nicaragua's history of both English and Spanish colonialism and North American military and economic interventions, these critiques have teeth. A number of women and men I interviewed during my research felt both empowered by these new identities and at the same time reported an increase in violent attacks against them because of their perceived status as "*homosexual*" or "*lesbiana*." Where hate crimes against non-heterosexual people were rare or non-existent in the past, they appear to be on the increase at the same time that new sexual identities are creating greater visibility for same-sex attracted people in Nicaragua.

Telenovelas and the entertainment politics of sexuality

Conveying particular images and narratives on television has become increasingly important to Nicaraguan activists hoping to create a greater range of cultural models around gender and sexuality. *El Sexto Sentido* (the Sixth Sense), a television show in Nicaragua, produced by a local feminist NGO, quickly became the most popular TV show when it began in 2001. According to poll research, 70 percent of Nicaraguan viewers were tuned in to *Sexto Sentido* every Sunday afternoon. Part soap opera, part sitcom, *Sexto* focuses on the lives of three young women and three young men. Funding proposals to USAID (United States Aid for International Development) hailed the show as a Nicaraguan version of the US-produced sitcom *Friends*. While the show's format may have a US legacy, during interviews people unanimously agreed, "We *love* the show because it is *pura Nicaragüense*." That is, it is "really Nicaraguan," in comparison to the usual TV programming from Mexico, Colombia, Brazil, and the United States. Shot on location with small digital cameras, and using colloquial expressions and jokes from around Nicaragua, the show is an intimately local production.

One of the show's producers, Iliana*, described the program as "pro-social entertainment TV," meant for Nicaraguan youth and their families. *Sexto* is a didactic show but definitely entertaining. It addresses reproductive health, gender and family violence, sexism, racism, prejudice against disabled individuals, negative stereotyping of rural peoples, and *heterosexismo* (heterosexism). The show features gay and lesbian characters and each episode focuses on the dynamics around romance, acceptance, and friendship—all of which are meant to instigate conversations on Nicaraguan street corners and family's living rooms. The show itself is a vehicle for stories out of which people spin more stories, providing a place for reflection and unfolding discussions around tolerance, identity, sexuality, desire, and behavior. Given the controversial topics, including abortion (illegal in Nicaragua), unintended pregnancies, and homosexuality—there is plenty for families and youth to talk about.

As an outreach device, the TV show is proving itself effective locally. If only a certain segment of the Nicaraguan population was privy to homosexuality as an identity in the past, these ideas are now available to everyone in the country. The show is inexpensive and delivers potent messages on the local level. But the show also has international appeal and is being screened in other Central American countries. The TV show draws together transnationally available concepts of human rights and other burgeoning universalisms, such as gay and lesbian identity, as well as the more established discourse of women's rights.

Carlos's political history and his comments at the beginning of this chapter prefigure, in an uncanny way, much of what would occur in Nicaragua over the next twenty years. His experience foreshadows the reciprocal relationships between one era's socialist aspirations and a next generation of identity-based movements for social justice that have taken media and technology as their platform. In the heat of the cold war, Nicaragua was a decisive battleground in global struggles around political economic systems and a thorn in the side of the US. Now, it is a place where dynamic and innovative approaches to sexual rights are being played out not only in the form of street protest, but perhaps more importantly, on Nicaraguan televisions. For advocates hoping to change the sexual culture of Nicaragua, media has a powerful potential to transform the way people think and talk about sexuality. In many ways, what we might call an "erotiscape" concerning sexual rights in Nicaragua is emerging now, both on the street and on the screen.

49 Sexuality in times of war

Gilbert Herdt

In the early 1930s Freud and Einstein exchanged letters that debated the critical question of their time: Why war? The exchange of ideas between two of the greatest minds of the century foreshadowed a terrible and dark reminder of the roots of war—atrocities and terrorism committed in the name of national service, and the deadly results of human suffering with which all people are faced today. Why do humans wage war? Their passionate public letters, coming in the early 1930s between the two great wars, continue to haunt everyone who is concerned with the world order.

These great minds did not, however, question the impact of war upon sexuality and the exaggeration of masculinity, or the role that rape and sexual violence plays in the humiliation of groups and nations at war. Gender roles are very much a part of the fabric of society, and thus implicated in the social and material conditions of warfare. Yet the question of how war distorts gender and exaggerates male prowess, conquest, prostitution, and rape as a tool of war were absent from the discussion of how war effects gender, sexual intimacy, and bodily integrity.

Those questions were to await a new century with its own growing recognition of sexuality as a human right. Today, there is an emerging international recognition that war has helped produce prostitution or commercial sex throughout world history. Moreover, rape is increasingly defined as a tool of war, which ought to be viewed as a crime against humanity—as defined by the International Criminal Court. This recognition is nascent and only beginning to seep into the understanding of how gender expectations impact the creation and continuance of war and the valorization of the kind of masculine personalities that often brutalize "the enemy" in sexual ways, including sexual violence and rape.

Domestic violence and sexual coercion, which is often hidden, haunts soldiers and their families—extending the war abroad to a war at home. In the ranks of all branches of the US military, homophobia continues to operate and influence judicial decisions and the operation of policies such as "Don't Ask, Don't Tell." Sexual commerce, trafficking, and prostitution typically follow in the wake of military deployments. Sexually transmitted disease epidemics have often erupted in the aftermath of war. Warfare and militarization in the United States, Latin America, and around the world have undermined human dignity and rights—especially women's rights. The integrity of women and children's bodies has been sacrificed as rape continues to be a weapon of warfare even today. As militarization increases around the globe, we should be concerned about the physical and psychological impact that this will have upon all people's sexuality.

Warfare and sex commerce

Wherever armies go, it has been observed, there follows sexual commerce and the worst forms of rape, sexual abuse, and prostitution. Women and children are the targets; however, boys and men have also been used as a means to humiliate enemies—bringing local authority to its knees. Objectifying the enemy as a sexual target and utilizing rape as a means to accomplish humiliation of "the other" have been used by warriors and armies since ancient times. We need only remember that as the Roman Empire expanded to encompass the Known World, prostitutes (some of them sexually enslaved or colonized as spoils of war) followed the Roman legions to the far corners of the empire, sickening or dying there. Likewise, the British Empire, with its Victorian double standard, was to treat colonized local peoples in India, South Africa, and Borneo as effeminate or less than masculine savages—sexual chattel that would produce bastards in the *Heart of Darkness*—never to mix with the gentile legal wife and heirs at home and unlikely to see the mother country and enjoy its privileges back in England.

Social scientists know only too well the dreadful impact of war upon society and culture, but until recently we did not study its pernicious impact within the military. As Margaret Mead once wrote in *Sex and Temperament in Three Primitive Societies* (1935), war may be natural, but the aggression and violence necessary to execute is not. A masculinity that is ruthless and aggressive requires ritual and mythology to mold men into phallic warriors able to maim and kill in the hand to hand combat, which was prevalent before the modern period.

My work among the Sambia of New Guinea has continually demonstrated that men must be trained and molded into warriors; it is not a natural outcome. Even then, some men do not have the personality capable of killing upon demand. Warfare serves, however, to magnify gender roles, twisting men and women into the extreme and exaggerated stereotypes we recognize in mythology around the world; these exaggerated stereotypes are also familiar to anyone who has seen Hollywood movies.

Consider the Sambia mythology of the Great Man/War leader. A Sambia man was trained in the men's house in secret for years through initiation rituals; this compression of gender training produced the desired effect. Rape was a constant threat in Sambia society; women and children were ever poised for constant attack from enemies, for the Sambia lived with the sense that "a war is going on." A young man was not accepted as *a real* man until he had stolen another man's wife and traveled with a war raiding party into the neighboring enemy tribe to kill the men. There, he was required to ruin their gardens and destroy their village, carrying away as many women as possible as political spoils.

Margaret Mead once referred to women abducted in the Admiralty Islands off the coast of New Guinea as "prostitutes" who serviced the men's house that had taken them. The film *Guardians of the Flutes* (British Broadcasting Corporation, 1993), titled after my first book, depicts a Sambia war leader who aggressively turns his pig's tusk nose plug so that its tusks point upward on his face. When Sambia men went to battle, the tusk signified how their penises were erect as well—a direct challenge to the masculinity of their enemies. It was said that such an image struck terror into the hearts of their opponents.

Military sexual conquest and modernity

In the last century the dark and ugly large-scale impact of war upon sexuality repeatedly appeared before and during World War II. Consider the Japanese invasion in the 1930s of Nanking, China, in what was to become known as the "rape of Nanking"—a dreadful, brutalized, sexual assault on women and children. It is an episode of military sexual conquest that remains a terrible sore point in Sino-Japanese relations today. Remember also the parallel sexual conquest of Korea by the Japanese, and the creation of Korean "comfort women," whose shame and anger even today remains a matter of bitter and painful international dispute.

The Nazi's sexual humiliation of women was part of a systemic attitude of profound violation of all human dignity and rights that led to the horrible abuses suffered by women and homosexuals in concentration camps. Cruel sexual commerce was therein created, one of the most shameful chapters of the Holocaust. When the Allies liberated Western Europe, local village and townspeople were the first to attack the women who had sexually mingled with the Germans for favors including food. Before the Allies got to the scene, local people's rage and shame was vented upon these local women. They were dragged into the streets and stripped naked, their heads were shaved, and they were further physically abused. Exile was often the only means of escape for these women; in one sense they were double victims of warfare.

Rape remains a weapon of choice in war today. During the long and bitter warfare in Bosnia-Herzegovina, it has been reported that thousands of women and children, including boys, were raped by enemies. Military conquest seemed to invite this horrific violation of bodies. Today, women and children are reportedly being raped on a large-scale basis in the Congo, as civil war and international political and economic circumstances create the setting for the most terrible forms of sexual assault and murder.

American military sexualization

These examples from other countries and other historical periods should not lead us away from examining our own specific American history and policies regarding the impact of war upon sex. Warfare has continuously exaggerated gender in our society, especially the performance of masculinity—creating the awful extremes of idealized women and men—even comic-book-like parodies of intimacy, romance, sexual intimidation, conquest, and rape, all of which are familiar in the movies, mass media, and Internet today.

The beautiful and tragic opera *Madame Butterfly* by Italian composer Puccini is based on a nineteenth-century myth about the sexual colonization of the East and exotic others by the West—in this case the United States, in its "opening" of Japan. Captain Pinkerton, a young and swashbuckling American officer in the US Navy, has a sexual liaison with a beautiful Japanese woman, who is both well born and then fallen. Butterfly falls in love with the handsome sea captain, but he abandons her and her offspring and refuses to take responsibility for his actions. When Pinkerton returns with his proper American wife, Butterfly realizes how he has betrayed her and her ensuing shame is so great that only ritual suicide (*seppuku*) can end the abuse and thus salvage her honor. Here is but the first "modern" example of a general process: wherever the US military has gone, sexual commerce, rape, and sexual spoils have followed in its wake.

American armed forces were central to the epidemic of syphilis created in World War I and World War II. The spread of the disease was controlled by quarantine and the internment of prostitutes, thus denying their rights. In the decades to follow, sexual liaisons between Americans and Japanese during the postwar occupation of Japan, and the sexual commerce with Korean women during and after the Korean War in the 1950s were but harbingers of a global phenomenon to come.

The Vietnam War inaugurated an era of massive consumption of sexual services. The French initiated the creation of a huge sex industry in Thailand and other corners of Southeast Asia. There, French and then American men who took "R and R" in these exotic places were provided with a sexual outlet sanctioned by the authorities and implicitly financed by the US government through the salaries and transport of men routinely sent for "relaxation." This was part and parcel of the gender and sexual climate of the times, which pitted the "good guys" against the "bad guys"—often framed as a struggle against Communism. Take note that many of the offspring of these sexual unions, occupied bodies in Germany, Japan, Korea, and Southeast Asia, were treated as illicit, expendable "nonhumans." Americans often chose not to take responsibility for these children, just as Pinkerton had done in *Madame Butterfly*.

The sexual victimization and exploitation that occurred in brothels and sex clubs in Southeast Asia foreshadowed much worse to come—the sex tourism industry on a gigantic scale and its dependence upon poverty and even the kidnapping of young women from Burma and other countries in the 1990s. Women and young males brought into this sex trade were exposed to a human suffering made worse by the horrors of the AIDS epidemic swiftly spreading among sex workers. The effort today to teach about safer sex and to provide condoms for barrier protection against HIV and other STDs has to some extent been successful. However, the legacy of sexual tourism remains. Granted, this sex trade is in part a form of income and commerce for individuals and the countries involved. Nevertheless, it cannot be denied that this form of sexuality was created in the context, at least partially, of war and poverty and the effects of countries that failed to take responsibility for the results of their actions during war.

In the early twenty-first century it is ours to ask: Not why war? But why sexual conquest and rape in war? How can we put a stop to rape and the dreadful impact of war upon gender roles and sexual intimacy; including the creation of unwanted pregnancy, HIV/AIDS, and the wholesale sexual conquest of people that violates human rights and bodily integrity?

One of the keys is for all nations, including the United States, to recognize the twenty-first-century principle that rape is a crime of war. The United States has refused to accept this ruling. Gender and sexuality are too fragile to resist the intimidations of war and warrior training, and the American experience is no different. Brutality wrought by sexual conquest must stop. The use of forced prostitution and sexual slavery must stop. It is time for all of us who regard human rights as inviolable to insist upon a higher standard by which all nations outlaw sexual violence during peace and war and forbid the use of rape as a weapon of warfare. The United States ought to act upon the values that we purport to uphold by ratifying the International Criminal Court's Rome statute that enforces rape as a crime of war. There is no single act that will better signal our commitment to ending sexual violence and sexual exploitation in times of war.

50 Revealing the soldier

Peacekeeping and prostitution

Paul Higate

The links between the presence of peacekeepers and the growth of prostitution in UN mission areas has received increased attention in recent years. In addition, and perhaps more disturbingly, a series of sexual violations against women and girls by peacekeepers have also been documented across the range of UN peacekeeping missions.

These include the rape and murder of a twelve-year-old Kosovo-Albanian girl by a UN peacekeeper, the alleged rape of a ten-year-old Congolese girl by a Moroccan peacekeeper, the production of a pornographic film through the exploitation of a local woman by an Irish peacekeeper in Eritrea, and the high-profile exchange of goods vital for survival—such as food and material for shelter—for sex by humanitarian workers and peacekeepers in refugee camps in Guinea, Liberia, and Sierra Leone.

These and numerous other reports appear to point to the flourishing of an aggressive sexuality that fails to discern between minors and adults and that may even result in the rape and death of vulnerable female, and in some cases male civilians (such as occurred in Somalia) in conflict and post-conflict societies. We must critically evaluate the sexual dynamics of peacekeeping contexts and at the same time recognize the valuable work that the UN continues to undertake.

The existence of prostitution and sexual violation of minors in mission areas is all the more shocking since it involves personnel in whom considerable trust is placed. To many, the peacekeeper is synonymous with security and a sense of reassurance and professional commitment. This imagery is powerfully influenced by the media whose dominant representation of peacekeepers accords with the popular psyche in that they are typically presented as blue-bereted saviors of the war-torn citizenry. Television pictures of peacekeepers holding babies, handing sweets to children, and disarming militia foreground the softer and more positive side of mainly (military) men trained in the use of force.

The peacekeeper comes to symbolically represent the conscience of the international community, and in this way we may project onto them our hopes and desires for societies that have endured genocide, massacres, and interminable suffering. It is hardly surprising then that perception of peacekeeper-identity tends toward a professional uni-dimensionality, as this links with their official activities in the public realm. Given this dominant portrayal, it is unsurprising that reactions to reports of sexual violations by peacekeepers invoke despair and outrage and are rooted in a sense that these men have reneged on their moral duty in the most pernicious of ways. The actions of a number of these peacekeepers (thought of as "GIs," "squaddies," and "troops") toward women and girls begins to fit with a commonly held view that military hypermasculinity can impact negatively on particular members of a vulnerable civilian population.

Making military men

In order to begin to illuminate the factors that appear to dispose some peacekeepers to sexually exploit local women and girls, it is necessary to consider the dominant form of masculinity that is developed in the military. Broadly speaking, this serves to create and reinforce a firm distinction between the genders and is expressed in the celebration of an aggressive, and frequently misogynist, heterosexuality. This gendered divide takes a multitude of forms though typically treats the feminine as the inferior "other." The feminine is linked to poor performance, inadequacy, incompetence, and weakness. In offsetting masculinity against femininity, the former is celebrated as all that the latter is not. Yet, the military is not unique in its gendered ideology; rather, it represents a microcosm and amplification of civilian institutions including the police force and fire service. It remains the case that, as Joshua Goldstein argues, soldiers show an "almost universal preoccupation with sex," and that, particularly in times of war (and we might add, in times of peace), "most soldiers were ready to have sexual intercourse with any woman wherever they could."

Discussions about sex, images of sex, constant references to sex, and the sexual conquest of women are relayed graphically and frequently, functioning as the lynchpin upon which the soldiering profession turns. As the Canadian sociologist Deborah Harrison has suggested: "the members of especially macho [military] units celebrate their shared maleness by objectifying women, viewing pornography films and joking about making women the targets of violence." In order to develop military masculine sexuality, it is necessary for recruits to be exposed to an intense period of military socialization.

This process starts prior to enlistment with the idea of the archetypal warrior figure whose tough, invulnerable, and sexually potent persona is revered and celebrated throughout popular and other cultural mediums. Military recruits—in the main adolescent men—are already likely to be familiar with this aspect of soldiering from comic books and movies. Undoubtedly, many are motivated by the possibility that enlistment into the military will encourage the development of heterosexual virility through the organization's association with the "making of men." Perhaps a number of enlistees are subconsciously seeking out an environment conducive to fostering and attaining manhood that many of their peers and family will quietly celebrate.

One aspect of military indoctrination that may also be of relevance to understanding the nature of gendered relations in, and around, military installations is the ability for troops to dehumanize the enemy or the "other." Women, as a socially subordinate group, are frequent victims of this othering as the Mai Lai massacre, in which US troops butchered women and girls in a Vietnamese village, graphically demonstrates. When a macho culture promoting aggressive heterosexuality is combined with strategies designed to strip away the humanity of others, the possibilities for sexual violation of women and girls increase significantly and have been powerfully portrayed in the movie *Casualties of War*.

Variations on a theme: sexualities in the military

When focusing on the sexuality of military personnel, it is important to recognize the heterogeneity of the organization in terms of the existence of sexualities that come into sharp focus when subject to a more fine-grained analysis. This is significant, not only in respect of the more obvious distinction between homosexuality and heterosexuality (a more liberal approach to homosexuality in the military has emerged on both side of the Atlantic in recent years) and the growing proportion of military women, but also in terms of how masculinity is performed. It is important to note that not all military men use prostitutes or rape, for example. Further, in discussing peacekeeping troops, there should be an acknowledgment that nationalities may differ in how they manage gendered relations together with the extent to which they view women and girls as subordinate. It is all too easy to work with a monolithic understanding of military masculine heterosexuality that may limit policy responses intended to modify the more destructive variants of peacekeeper's impact on gendered relations. In addition to rank, there may also be differences in the ways that Military Observers (commissioned officers) manage their sexuality when contrasted with the heterosexual performances of members of the contingent personnel (non-commissioned ranks who guard UN assets). The former may exercise discretion in their sexual liaisons, while contingent soldiers tend to celebrate their heterosexuality in public in bars and brothels, easily identifiable in their uniform and large groups.

Cynthia Enloe has written about the military's support of prostitution in close proximity to its bases or in zones designated for the rest and recreation of officers and men. Throughout the extensive history of the close relationship between camp-following women and the military, the psychological and health interests of military men have been prioritized over those of the women whose role it is to provide a vital sexual outlet, while being under medical surveillance by the military authorities. This control and monitoring of militarized prostitutes has involved oppressive practices, including the use of degrading examinations through which their part in the spreading of sexually transmitted diseases has been highlighted, while the role of the men in this process has been ignored. The direct and unapologetic involvement of the military in prostitution lies in its belief systems that turn on a particular understanding of male sexuality.

To deny their men this sexual "safety valve" for a natural and barely controllable sex drive is to court serious problems, in which aggressive heterosexuality might prove dysfunctional. According to the military, denial of sex could result in a significant diminution in combat effectiveness as, in the absence of heterosexual activity, military men are unable to affirm all aspects of their warriorhood. Unscientific theories abound concerning testosterone levels and potential for aggression in respect of regular sexual intercourse, though there is little credible empirical evidence to support such a proposition. More disturbingly, so far as the military are concerned, is the possibility that men who are denied heterosexual contact, born of sheer desperation, will seek out homosexual liaisons with soldier colleagues. In this scenario it is envisaged that the military masculine "glue" cementing unit cohesion is likely to melt away, rendering impotent the now feminized fighting force. Thus, male sexuality in the military is akin to a truck whose brakes have failed. The best that can be hoped for is to steer it onto the correct highway; alternative routes are bound to result in disaster.

Exchanges of sharp inequality: peacekeepers and prostitution

In contemporary debates the question of prostitution divides commentators. The two extreme positions are represented by the notion that either all prostitution represents violence to women, or that women should be free to choose what they do with their bodies, seeing commercial sex as a form of sexual labor. Military thinking errs toward the latter position, and the frequent retort that poverty-stricken women are gaining financially from their interactions with peacekeepers is used to obscure the harsh realities of survival sex work. Many women and girls are forced into this form of income generation when faced with life and death circumstances for themselves and their families. Another argument made by the broad spectrum of prostitute clients—including military men—is that the women are "very active" in attracting their custom. The argument is made that because prostitutes "come on to you readily . . . and tell you that you are handsome," it is the woman, not the peacekeeper, who is responsible for the exchange. In this way peacekeepers are able to cast themselves as "helpless victims" with a biologically powerful sex drive that prostitutes "exploit."

There has been rather less discussion, at least in terms of those who might be described as military apologists, for the wide-scale existence of prostitution across the unique and frequently dysfunctional context of the peacekeeping mission. The post-conflict environment is one in which gendered relations are heavily distorted, and peacekeeper's involvement with prostitutes represents an exchange of fundamental financial inequality. For example, in terms of sharp financial disparity, in the MONUC mission in the Democratic Republic of Congo (DRC), the Mission Subsistence Allowance for UN peacekeeper Military Observers and some other UN civilian personnel is $138 per day, whereas the average *annual* income per head of Congolese citizen is $100. Such inequalities fuel the commodification of women and girls, many of whom bear the full brunt of conflict and—as was witnessed during the Balkan War—are raped as a key strategy designed to weaken the enemy's morale. A number of these rapes may result in pregnancy and the birth of babies who then place an additional burden on an already traumatized survivor of sexual violation. Many of these women become locked into a cycle of prostitution because of pressure to support a young family and facilitated by the damage to the mother's self-esteem; she may become resigned to meeting the sexual demands of UN clients. These factors, along with the age of consent and of marriage in both Sierra Leone and the DRC (currently fourteen years of age), contribute toward the cocktail of circumstances in which peacekeeper abuse is likely.

Zero tolerance

Kofi Annan, in responding to the scandals that continue to damage the UN's reputation, has called for a climate of "zero tolerance" with regard to the activities of peacekeeper violation of women and girls. However, there is ambiguity here as it is not entirely clear if prostitution is exempt from this strategy. In recent years across all peacekeeping missions, various Codes of Conduct have been formulated. The generic UN Blue Helmets Code of Conduct states that "peacekeepers will never commit any act that could result in sexual harm to members of the local population including women and children." Codes that reflect the particular conditions of the mission area (for example, the age of consent and marriage) have also been drawn up, along with the establishment of committees (for example, the UNAMSIL mission in Sierra Leone) whose terms of reference are specifically to monitor and highlight the issue of peacekeeper exploitation of women and girls. These codes use the language of "strict prohibition" of sexual contact with minors and of sexual exploitation of local women and girls by UN personnel, and they are uncompromising in their tone. They also suggest that *bona fide* relationships between peacekeepers and local women over age eighteen are acceptable.

Clearly, the codes are open to interpretation, not least because they are intended for a multinational audience who vary in their understandings of cultural norms and the nuances of language.

Ultimately, the UN is attempting to regulate the sexuality of its personnel and particularly its peacekeepers whose reputation for exploitation is of greater visibility than that of civilian staff. In this way, the UN stands at the interface of troop-contributing countries and concerned onlookers, who consider that prostitution in a post-war setting is unacceptable for personnel who have unique responsibilities. If it is considered that prostitution and exploitation are inseparable, then, for many, these codes are unworkable. Soldiering and prostitution—argued by some to be the "two oldest professions"—feed off one another and exist in a symbiotic relationship that can only be detached by resorting to, according to the military, oppressive practice, such as turning troop barracks into virtual prisons. If, however, prostitution is not considered as exploitation, then the codes have some chance of success and the masculinized culture of the UN retains a key outlet for certain elements of its personnel.

It would appear that the aggressive heterosexuality of a significant number of peacekeepers is somewhat unique. Yet in many ways, the activities of these men differ little from those of sex tourists, for example. UN peacekeepers encounter extreme inequality and vulnerable minors, similar to conditions found at many sex tourism destinations.

This should not be taken as a condemnation of the work of the UN, as undoubtedly its interventions over the years have proved crucial to the preservation of life and the creation of peace. However, the UN is caught between national militaries on which it depends for peacekeepers and demands by those deemed to be "outsiders" that they significantly temper the aggressive heterosexuality of these troops. One place to start, and here we add to a growing clamor for action of this sort, is for the perpetrators of sexual violation against women and girls to be brought to rapid and decisive justice. The impunity they currently enjoy sits closely with the notion that these men really are at the whim of a biological drive that can override their sense of moral duty.

51 "R and R" on a "hardship tour"

GIs and Filipina entertainers in South Korea

Sealing Cheng

Eddy* was a twenty-year-old GI who had heard a lot about cheap sex in Korea. By the time he arrived in the country, he felt compelled to try the "thirty-buck-a-trick" experience negotiated through a pimp on the street. He explained, "I had to do it. I have heard so much about it that I had to do it."

Eddy then spent the next six months of his time and money, buying drinks for women and hoping to find a girlfriend in one of the clubs. Many of his peers did the same. He finally gave up because, he said:

> It's not sincere. That's why I don't like it. A relationship with a "drinkie girl" is not normal. But it's just almost impossible to have a GI girl, there are about two (women) to every eight hundred men. We call it the "hateway" rather than the gateway. You have to fight so hard to get through it. And one day, I just decided that I couldn't take it anymore. Of course I feel lonely . . . Yes, there is the loneliness, but I can handle it.

The history of rest and relaxation

Prostitution has become synonymous with the rest and relaxation (R and R) industry for the US military abroad, particularly in East and Southeast Asia. Clubs for GIs have sprung up around US military camp towns in the Philippines, Japan, in particular Okinawa, Vietnam, and South Korea. These GI clubs are the progeny of a global network of US military bases formed for the containment of Communism and the preservation of US geopolitical interests. Recent reports of the trafficking of women from the Philippines and former Soviet countries to GI clubs in South Korea have fueled criticisms of the US military overseas.

South Korea—still technically at war with North Korea due to the legacy of the Korean War—remains one of the most heavily armed zones on earth. In 2001, 37,000 US military personnel are standing by for war on the Korean peninsula. For GIs, clubs around bases provide a welcome relief from work in the form of alcohol, music, and most importantly, women. For people working in the R and R industry, the GIs' desires and patronage are vital to their livelihood.

The profile of women entertaining GIs in Korea has changed significantly in the last decade. In the post-war years, Korean women worked in GI clubs and were dubbed

---

*Names changed to protect privacy.

with such derogatory terms as "Western whores" and "Western princesses." In the 1990s Korea's rapid economic advancement led to a shortage of Korean women willing to serve these American soldiers; the stigma and relatively low income made it a losing proposition for many Korean women. In order to fill the vacancies left by Korean women, women were imported from the "third world." Since the 1980s the Korean government has allowed for a limited number of cheap foreign laborers to take up the "3D" (dangerous, dirty, and difficult) jobs abandoned by Korean nationals. According to some Korean and Filipino activists, Filipino women have been "trafficked" to relieve the shortage of entertainers in military camp towns in South Korea (*kichich'on*) since 1996.

In the 1990s customer profiles changed. In addition to US military personnel, foreigners on business trips or working in nearby factories, as well as Koreans, now frequent the clubs. Korean men often visit the clubs because of the perceived exoticness of foreign women entertainers. With more spending power than GIs, coupled with often extravagant spending habits, Korean men have become an increasingly important source of revenue for *kichich'on* clubs.

The changing demographics in *kichich'on* clubs, at the level of patrons and workers, are impacted by the changing power relationship between the United States, Korea, and the Philippines. Even though US military domination continues in the Asian-Pacific region, US military forces have lost much of their economic sway. Korea has not only achieved greater economic independence from the United States, but has gained economic power in the region. Changing economic conditions have made it possible for Korea to invest in and import cheap labor from poorer countries such as the Philippines.

My fieldwork in two US military camp towns in South Korea, between 1998 and 2001, focused on how migrant Filipinas make sense of their lives as entertainers in GI clubs. I also set out to understand the meanings that GIs and Korean club owners attributed to their interactions with Filipina entertainers, and how these dynamics between individuals are embedded in the larger political economy of the Asian-Pacific region.

Many social science analyses of military prostitution have largely focused on the voice of women who perform sex work. For the most part, this body of literature has identified their oppression and suffering as a casualty of masculinist state projects, their prostituted bodies serving as a symbol of poor nations' dominated status. While this perspective accounts for the structural relationship between GIs and women entertainers, it does not provide insight into the everyday interactions between them. My perspective, here, adopts the rather unconventional method of introducing R and R industry in South Korea from the GIs' perspective.

Previous research has not paid much attention to GIs' experiences due in part to an ambivalent understanding of military servicemen in the eyes of middle-class America. In times of war, they are heroes, as seen in the media coverage of the Iraq War. In times of peace, they are mere hirelings of the military machinery who have failed to "make it" in American society. According to this stereotype, young American male soldiers are regarded as drunkards and sexual predators who, were it not for military discipline and their roles as warriors, would live on the margins of US society. Recent statistics from the US Department of Defense detailing the educational achievements and ethnic composition of active duty US military personnel show that although GIs do not rank in the top percentages of academic prowess, neither are they "rejects" of the education system. Overall, stereotypes about military personnel that configure GIs as mere dupes of the military machine do not account for the reality of military men and women. My position is that it is important to account for GIs' motives and emotions when considering the dynamics of sex work, military camps, and militarized territories.

GI clubs in Korea

A mission to Korea is, according to military categorization, a "hardship" tour. There is no government sponsorship for family members and most GIs live alone while overseas in Korea. The tour normally lasts for one year. The short duration of the assignment seems to justify the absence of programs to integrate GIs into the host country. There are no language skills training or briefing sessions on the social and cultural makeup of the country.

In this context the R and R facilities around US military bases become the main venue for American soldiers' off-post activities. What actually does the R and R in Korea offer?

The minute they step off the base, GIs find clubs where they come face to face with scantily clad Asian women—all of whom are eager to shower their attention on any man for the price of a drink. While some GIs go to clubs in groups to play pool or darts, a patron who arrives alone sends a clear message that he is in search of a woman. As soon as he enters a club, an entertainer will greet him and bring him to his table. A US$10 drink will buy him the company of a woman for a short while. (Some club owners set the time limit to twenty minutes.) Continual company requires his purchasing more drinks. A woman might just sit next to the customer, perform a provocative dance, or rub herself against the man's groin before requesting a drink. What a woman will do in exchange for drinks depends upon the customer, the club, the woman, and her need for drinks and remuneration on any particular day.

The euphoria men enjoy while they are being fawned over by women is, however, constantly at risk. A man's popularity declines or increases according to the hard cash he possesses. Low-ranking GIs, whose salaries are likewise low, are more likely to have short lived encounters with entertainers. High-ranking GIs with a handsome salary are able to buy multiple drinks for entertainers and coworkers; it is high-ranking GIs who are greeted most enthusiastically in the clubs. Those who refuse to buy the ladies drinks are often goaded with the name "Cheap Charlie." This directly challenges masculine pride, an assault that many young GIs find hard to endure. Many Filipinas are familiar with the power of such tactics to get more out of male customers.

Eddy, the twenty-one-year-old GI I interviewed, offered his own analysis of relationships with entertainers. "You see, they either make you feel pity for them, or make you feel special, or make you think that you are going to get something." Eddy's insight points to three common elements and tactics used by entertainers to gain customers' patronage: their own powerlessness, their customers' individuality, and the prospect of sex. These factors may operate separately, but more frequently they are combined to create an illusion of intimacy in *kichich'on* clubs.

In the context of *kichich'on* clubs, the "game of love" is an important element impacting the interactions between GIs and Filipinas. The "play" often has the potential to end in serious emotions. Mediated by the idioms of romantic love, money and sex become more than a matter of simple remunerative service transactions. In this context "boyfriends" have become synonymous with "customers"; "I love you" is a daily utterance and marriage proposals a weekly occurrence. Relationships in clubs are more complex than simply "male domination" and "female subordination"—the model put forward in most prostitution studies. This complexity is not readily revealed in many representations of the R and R industry; instead these complicated emotional and power-laden dynamics are often unambiguously categorized as "prostitution."

Filipina "entertainers"

The Filipinas who I interviewed were between the ages of seventeen and thirty-five, most of them in their early twenties. They were primarily from Manila, Pampanga, and the Laguna region of the Philippines. Only a few of them had worked in a club before coming to Korea. The women held E-6 visas (for "entertainers") and had one-year contracts. Before 1999 women arrived in Korea with the promise of a job as a waitress, dancer, or guest relations officer. Most of the women who have arrived since 2000 auditioned to be "entertainers," during which they posed in bikinis. Most women had a vague idea of what their jobs would entail but rarely did they understand from the outset the exact nature of their working conditions. Because of managers' attempts to conceal the truth of the working conditions and different kinds of club management, women were unsure of what they would encounter in the workplace. One thing they were aware of was the illegal nature of their migration and job. Because of the detour they took en route, via Hong Kong or Bangkok, and the lies they were taught to tell at immigration check points, women were well aware of their marginal legal status.

Upon arrival at the clubs, women's passports are often taken by club owners and a portion of their salaries are not paid until they leave Korea to prevent them from running away. The women are required to entertain GIs by encouraging them to buy as many $10 ladies' drinks as possible. The work day for women is sometimes as long as eighteen hours. Some women do not get a single day off for the entire year that they work in Korea, and some clubs require drink quotas that women must fulfill or they may be penalized. Entertainers receive only $2 for every $10 drink a customer buys for them. Some clubs with VIP rooms allow customers to bring a woman into the room for half an hour, providing that he buys four drinks for his female companion. A customer may also pay a "bar fine" in order to take a woman out of the club. According to the time of the month—bar fines are more expensive on pay days—and the length of time desired, bar fines range from $100 to $300. The women can expect to receive 20 percent of the money. Whatever happens in the VIP room, or on a "bar fine" outing, is negotiated between the woman and the customer.

"It's up to you," was the refrain commonly asserted by Filipina entertainers. The voluntary nature of their work was fundamental to the way many women articulated their professional lives. Katie* believed, for example, that "it's up to you" whether one prostituted oneself or not. She said that women could choose to run away—as she herself had done. Similarly, women who went on a "bar fine" with GIs might run off at any time, even before sex had been initiated. Janet* also said that "it's up to you" whether or not one performed oral sex for a customer in a VIP room. Many women did complain about pressure from club owners to increase sales. However, unlike many activists' claims that focus upon women's powerlessness, many entertainers I interviewed preferred to see themselves as autonomous agents, exercising control over their bodies and sexuality.

However, we should not underestimate the potential for abuse in the clubs. Because women are aware that they are engaged in an illegitimate trade, entertainers are reluctant to file complaints, fearing negative repercussions. Since their passports are held by club owners and their running away would immediately make them illegal aliens, it is only with tremendous courage, and usually following severe abuses, that the women leave the clubs. Many women are also reluctant to easily forgo their hard earned jobs in Korea, especially given the lack of employment opportunities in the Philippines.

Both local and international nongovernmental organizations (NGOs) identify these women as "victims of trafficking." Whether or not this is an accurate description, we should not be blind to the fact that women's structural vulnerability does not necessarily translate into personal powerlessness. In fact, entertainers' "weakness" may become their "weapons," prompting young American soldiers to answer their calls for "love" and support in the "game of love."

Recent developments

Increasingly, Filipina entertainers have fled the clubs and started to work in factories or live with their GI boyfriends—some in long-term relationships, others in a kind of "temporary marriage." In my last visit to a *kichich'on* in June 2003, I saw many more pregnant Filipinas around "American Alley" than I did three years previously. While a few of these relationships do end up in marriages, there is also a high degree of GIs abandoning their girlfriends, especially after she is pregnant, creating a difficult set of circumstances for the Filipina women and their children who are left behind. In some ways these Filipina women have become heiresses to both the lifestyles and the problems of their Korean predecessors in *kichich'on*.

The US military had planned on moving forces southwards, away from the border and Seoul. The fate of *kichich'on* in the north remains uncertain, while the major *kichich'on* in the south are celebrating the move. Military redeployment will likely be followed by a wave of foreign entertainers. Meanwhile, in June 2003 the Korean Ministry of Justice stopped issuing E-6 visas for foreign women entertainers. Because of the human rights violations implicit in this form of service, women entertainers' status has become a "diplomatic issue." While some may see this as a victory for the international anti-trafficking campaign, concerned NGOs and individuals worry that such a drastic move will only drive the flow of entertainers underground, increasing the incidence of abuse.

Understanding military prostitution—the case of South Korea

Our understanding of "military prostitution" and "trafficking" must be both more politicized and more personalized. On the one hand, beyond the role of the US military, other institutions allow for the abuses found in some GI clubs. These include local governments, government bureaucrats, club owners, and brokers (men and women who benefit in one way or another from the industry). Gender-based violence that has driven many women away from their homes to work overseas and a racialized nationalism that has subjected foreign women to greater discrimination impacts how entertainers are treated in Korean clubs. The international imbalance of power that has exacerbated individual countries' economic dependence on remittances has also impacted the lives of women who may feel compelled to undertake work as entertainers to support families back home. On the other hand, underlying this commercial exchange is the often romantic parable of discovery—the conquest of the US American (white) explorer, who is rewarded with an alien and exoticized lover who is both submissive and devoted. Notions of intimacy and love are commonly considered elusive, if not downright irrelevant, in the sexual services industry. Yet in the case of GI clubs, these transactions are often "personalized" and occur over a period of time—giving rise to a complexity that is difficult to untangle or grasp with a singular concept of "prostitution."

Index